Portrait *of* Healing

Curing in the Woods

Victoria E. Rinehart, EdD, RN, CNAA

Foreword by Garry Trudeau

Kathryn E. Dubois
Graphic Design and Layout

Editorial Assistance Provided by:
Mary Hotaling and Florence H. Wright

North Country Books, Inc.
311 Turner Street,
Utica, New York 13501

Portrait of Healing

©2002 Victoria E. Rinehart

Cover photo:

Second graduating class of the D. Ogden Mills Training School for Nurses in 1915
Miss Schwartz, Mrs. Smith, Miss Lake, and seated, Dr. Trudeau.
Courtesy of the Trudeau Institute Archives

Photo page xx:

Resting place of Trudeau Family beneath the tall pines at St. John's in the Wildnerness near St. Regis, New York
Courtesy of the Trudeau Institute Archives

Photo page 46:

Gated entrance into the Trudeau Sanatorium
Courtesy of the Trudeau Institute Archives

Photo page 106:

D. Ogden Mills Training School for Nurses at Trudeau Sanatorium
Courtesy of the Trudeau Institute Archives

Photo page 150:

Trudeau Statue with Flowers from Nurse's Graduation
Courtesy of the Trudeau Institute Archives

Back cover photo:

Dr. and Mrs. Trudeau with the 1915 graduating class of the D. Ogden Mills Training School for Nurses
Courtesy of the Trudeau Institute Archives

Library of Congress Cataloging-in-Publication Data
ISBN: 0-925168-83-1

North Country Books, Inc.
Publisher-Distributor
311 Turner Street
Utica, New York 13501

The cure for all ills and wrongs, the cares,
the sorrows and the crimes of humanity,
all lie in the one word 'love.'
It is the divine vitality that everywhere
produces and restores life.
*~**Lydia Maria Child***

For My Husband
Warren

For My Mother
Joan H. Evans

For My Daughters
Deb Sullivan and Tori Stevens

For Halle and Nate

And, of course, for Ben and Farley

Table of Contents

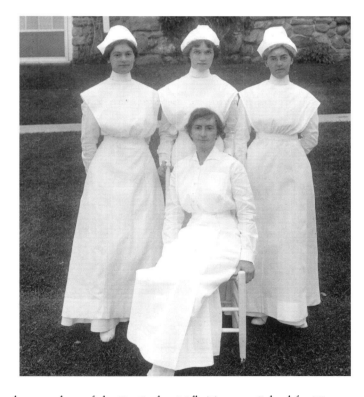

*Second graduating class of the D. Ogden Mills Training School for Nurses in 1915
Miss Schwartz, Mrs. Smith, Miss Lake, and seated, Miss O'Mally, Superintendent of Nurses.
Courtesy of the Trudeau Institute Archives*

I grew up in a company town, built upon a single industry, which one autumn day during my childhood simply ceased to be. Antibiotics had arrived, almost overnight, rendering the fresh-air cure completely irrelevant. The nurses and doctors were summoned, my grandfather gave a short speech, and then the cottages were boarded up, the wide porches with the magnificent views abandoned to the season's early snows. A photographer from Life came up to document the occasion, but he accidentally exposed his film in the sanatorium's X-ray lab, and by then the patients were gone, and with them a way of life. All that remained were tales of the countless consumptives who for 70 years had traveled to this hushed, gentle place to regain their health, and most of these would soon be forgotten.

This delightful book seeks to redress this loss to North Country heritage. By searching out the stories not just of the Adirondack Cottage Sanitarium's renowned founder, E.L. Trudeau, but also of the patients and the caregivers who served them so well, Victoria Rinehart not only humanizes the sanatorium story, but also reminds us just how original, even radical, the fresh-air treatment of tuberculosis was for its day. In 1884, the year the first cure cottage was built in Saranac Lake, medical knowledge about contagious disease was surprisingly limited, often drifting into outright superstition (indeed, it was shocking to learn from one patient's account that as late as 1948, the windows on the TB wards at New York Hospital were still being kept closed to prevent cross-ventilation). Edward Trudeau's key insight was that ample portions of fresh air, good food and rest could be curative, that the body would do wonders to restore itself if certain conditions of physical well-being and psychological and spiritual uplift could be maintained.

Some critics later observed that this was no insight at all, that Trudeau was not really "curing" people, but rather simply allowing them to cure themselves. This, of course, is the dirty, little secret of much of modern medicine — that the vast majority of our maladies will usually retreat on their own without the slightest assist from anything but our own remarkable ability to heal ourselves — clearly a component of our evolutionary success. In this respect, my great-grandfather's work foreshadowed our current era's holistic movement, with its faith in natural approaches to healing. Stress-reduction, body massage, occupational therapy, proper diet — these were not the invention of California ashrams, but were rather the restorative strategies carefully devised by the pioneers of the turn-of-the-century sanatorium movement.

For a few years after its gates were closed, the Trudeau Sanatorium, locally known as the "San", remained vacant, inhabited only by squirrels and ghosts, and the young boy who bicycled down Trudeau Road into the warren of graceful buildings that formed the town of Trudeau, New York, could scarcely comprehend why his ubiquitous name had come to stand for so much for so many. There was the beautiful bronze statue of the great healer, situated on the hillside just below the main road, but surrounded as it was by forlorn, decommissioned cottages, his legacy was not obvious to me. ELT was a general in a war that had been largely forgotten, and even today, as TB rages around the world, still slaughtering millions in its wake, our strategies for resisting it owe little to the cure chairs and sputum jars of sanatorium life.

But Trudeau's great talent, I now understand, was for hope — a commodity in short supply during the worst years of the White Plague. People came to Saranac Lake to cure, not to die, and that was new. Indeed, most of them did recover, and the experience was transformative, compelling many of them to stay on and virtually all of them to regard their days at the San as some of the happiest of their lives. This book, lovingly researched and gracefully presented, helps us understand how such abundant affection could be possible.

~Garry Trudeau

To Dr. and Mrs. Edward Livingston Trudeau

Thank you

May your kindness always live on in others.
It is my hope that every person who reads this book
Will extend just one act of "Trudeauism" to another.

Profits from the sale of this book will be donated to:

The Trudeau Institute
Biomedical Research Laboratory
Saranac Lake, New York

~VER

Acknowledgements

It is impossible to give adequate thanks to all the people who have helped, in so many different ways, with this project. To my husband, Warren, who endured my frequent trips to the Adirondacks and whose love and endless words of encouragement sustained me. His patience and understanding were unwavering. To my mother, whose excitement over the daily manuscript readings energized me. Love and thanks to my daughters, Deb and Tori. Just knowing they are there fills my heart with joy. To my grandchildren, Halle and Nate, special thanks. Thinking about them during the moments of discouragement helped me to refocus on what really matters. To Ben and Farley, my bearded collies, who literally dragged me away from the computer every afternoon promptly at five demanding their supper. And to Fran Davis, my good friend and Adirondack neighbor, whose enthusiasm over this project continually recharged my commitment to finish.

I would like to offer special thanks and appreciation to Garry Trudeau for writing the forward to this book. That his words should introduce the book that brings the good works of his great-grandfather back to life completes the cycle of history and touches me beyond words.

Very deep gratitude is extended to the three deans of nursing that I have had the privilege of working under while at the State University of New York Institute of Technology at Utica/Rome (SUNYIT). To Ellen Coher who eliminated so many obstacles while I completed my doctoral degree at Teacher's College, Columbia University. Special thanks to Elizabeth Kellogg Walker who insisted I take the sabbatical in order to complete this project and to my current dean, Jeannine Muldoon, whose support and words of encouragement have been unending. Also my sincere thanks to Jackie Coughlan, Associate Librarian at SUNYIT, for her ability to retrieve just about any resource I needed, to the nursing faculty who helped to pick up my workload while I was out on academic leave, to Nancy Rickard for her hours of transcription, and to Mary Ann Randazzo, just because. Great appreciation is also extended to Peter J. Cayan, President of SUNYIT. As a seasonal resident of Saranac Lake, he has been a very useful source of information. His sustained interest and multifaceted assistance with this project have been invaluable.

This project could not have been completed without the assistance of the many nurses who cured and worked at Trudeau Sanatorium and other patient "graduates" whose willingness to offer their words and memories added so much richness and credibility to Portrait of Healing. Sincere thanks to Bea Sprague Edward, Jean Gage, Ethyl Healy, Mel Levine, Ann Lewis, Peg McLaughlin, Jen McNeil, Emma Montalbine, Rose and Irving Muschlin, and Cathy Pendergast. I am deeply indebted to both Anne Irene Remis and Lilo Levine for their respective contributions to Chapters 2 and 3. The poignant reminiscences of their TB experience offer a touching close-up perspective of what life was really like on the inside of Trudeau Sanatorium. And for the nurses and past patients whom I was unable to reach in time, hopefully this book has been able to capture the essence of your experiences as well. Deepest gratitude also to Ursula Trudeau who steered me in the right direction more than once!

This book would not have been possible without the archives of the Trudeau Institute Biomedical Research Laboratory and the untiring help of Linda Auclair, Librarian, and Susan Cooper, Director of Institutional Advancement, who went out of their way to offer me unlimited access to all the available archives and records. Special thanks also to Michele Tucker, Curator of the Adirondack Room, Saranac Lake Free Library, who spent many long hours patiently emailing me very large graphic files.

Thanks also to Jeanine Young-Mason for her incredible words of wisdom; and to Martie Gullion, Beverly Ianuzi, Peggy O'Shea, Reggie Smith, Wendy Poole, and Kaffie McCollough who personify support. And, of course, I will always be indebted to my students who for so many years have been encouraging me to write this book. Their intellect, humor, and unending quest for knowledge have kept alive my love of teaching.

Also sincere appreciation to Mary Hotaling. Her vast knowledge of the history of Saranac Lake and editorial assistance have been invaluable. Deep gratitude also to Florence Wright for her multifaceted help with indexing, sharing of her postcard collection, and numerous helpful editorial comments. And finally, there simply are not enough words to thank my niece, Katie Dubois, the incredibly gifted graphics designer who performed magic on every page in this book. There was no challenge too great for her. Without her sense of humor and calming influence, this book would never have been completed. And to all the people long gone whose words are quoted in this book, thank you for your contributions in helping to record the history of this memorable institution.

~Victoria E. Rinehart

It was neither sleet nor snow, just something in between. It was the kind of cold that gets into your bones and hangs on tight. On a dreary Saturday afternoon in early November, I was walking along the streets of Saranac Lake, New York, conducting a class with six shivering nursing students. As much as I wanted to escape into the warm comfort of my car and begin the three-hour trip home to Utica, New York, I couldn't leave until the class was over. At some point, during the course of that cold afternoon, the idea for this book began to germinate.

One of the courses that I teach at SUNYIT is an undergraduate nursing research course. Perhaps due to boredom, my students would stare back at me with glazed expressions on their faces during the content on historical research. I obviously was not reaching them. How could I bring something old to life for them and give it meaning?

All my life I have traveled through Saranac Lake on the way to vacation in Lake Placid. My mother often talked about a friend from Rome, New York, whose mother, Bessie Comstock, contracted tuberculosis, cured, and later died in Saranac Lake. Betty Mooney subsequently wrote the book, *In the Shadow of the White Plague*, which told of her mother's experience in Saranac Lake. As a result of hearing Betty's story from my mother and reading her book, the houses that lined the streets of Saranac Lake, all with their little cure porches attached, always fascinated me. I wanted to know more.

It was the reading of Phil Gallos' excellent history, *Cure Cottages of Saranac Lake*, which gave me the idea for the class. On a whim, although I had never met Phil, I called and asked if he would meet my six students and me to provide a walking tour of the cure cottages. Much to my delight, he obliged. During that bone-chilling afternoon, Phil mesmerized all of us with his description of the cure cottage history of Saranac Lake. Mary Hotaling, director of Historic Saranac Lake, later joined us to provide a tour of the old grounds of Trudeau Sanatorium currently owned by the American Management Association.

History of a time long gone from the area was being brought to life that afternoon. Despite the cold, my students never once retreated into that distant place where students go when they are bored. But as eloquently as both Phil and Mary talked about that time in history, a piece was missing. Where were the stories of the doctors and nurses who had cured, studied, and practiced at Trudeau Sanatorium? And where were the stories about other patients, who had received the medical and nursing care by those lucky enough to have survived the great white plague of tuberculosis and, in so doing, felt the need to stay on at the sanatorium in order to help others?

This book will tell those stories. But they cannot be told without first describing the man who made Trudeau Sanatorium possible and the unique world of healing that he created on the side of Mt. Pisgah in the little village of Saranac Lake.

The Disease

Tuberculosis, also called the Great Killer, the White Plague, consumption, or phthisis, is an infectious disease caused by the bacilli *Mycobacterium tuberculosis*. It can affect several organs of the human body, including the brain, the kidneys, and the bones; but, most commonly, it affects the lungs (pulmonary tuberculosis). The primary or first phase of the infection usually lasts for several months. During this period, the body's natural defenses (immune system) resist the disease, and a fibrous capsule or tubercle that develops around the area walls in most or all of the bacteria. Before the initial attack is over, a few bacteria may escape into the bloodstream and be carried elsewhere in the body where they are again walled in. In many cases, the disease never develops beyond this latent or incipient phase. If, however, the immune system fails to stop the infection, and it is left untreated, the disease may progress to the second or active phase where the germ multiplies rapidly and destroys the tissues of the lungs (or the other affected organ). On the average, people infected with *M. tuberculosis* have a ten percent chance of developing active TB at some point in their lives.

As the bacilli spread to new sites, the body's defense system will kill many of the bacilli. In this process, however, immune cells and local tissue will die along with the bacilli. This process causes the formation of granulomas whose cheese-like centers form a place where the bacilli may survive. Early symptoms of active TB include weight loss, weakness, loss of appetite, chills, fever, and night sweats.

As more lung tissue is destroyed, causing the granulomas to enlarge, cavities in the lungs may develop and break into the larger airways called bronchi. Most likely this terminology gave rise to the term "breaking down" with TB that was so often used in the early 1900s. This break can cause a large number of bacilli to escape into the air when a patient coughs. Ultimately the progression of the disease will cause the granulomas to liquefy. This new medium produces an environment that is favorable for multiplication and further spread of the bacilli. At this point, the symptoms may worsen and include chest pain and cough. If a blood vessel becomes eroded, coughing of blood or hemorrhage may develop.

The TB germ is carried on droplets in the air and can enter the body through the airway. A person with active pulmonary tuberculosis can spread the disease by coughing or sneezing. The process of "catching" tuberculosis involves two stages: first, a person has to become infected; second, the infection has to progress to disease. Active disease is more likely in an individual whose immune system is compromised because of aging, HIV, malnutrition, injection drug use, and use of chemotherapy for treatment of cancer.

Tuberculosis was responsible for killing fourteen percent of the human race in the 1800s. Even by the 1940s, tuberculosis was killing more people than any other contagious disease. Currently, the registered number of new cases of TB worldwide roughly correlates with economic conditions: the highest incidences are seen in those countries of Africa, Asia, and Latin America with the lowest gross national products. The World Health Organization estimates that of the eight million people who get TB every year, ninety-five percent live in developing countries. One-third of the world's population is infected with TB. An estimated three million people die from TB every year.

A great influence in the rising TB trend is HIV infection. As previously stated, chances are only ten percent that immunocompetent people infected with *M. tuberculosis* will fall sick in their lifetimes, but among those with HIV, ten percent will develop active TB every year.

A final factor contributing to the resurgence of TB is the emergence of multi-drug resistance. Drug resistance in TB occurs as a result of *tubercle bacillus* mutations. These mutations are not dependent upon the presence of the drug. Exposed to a single effective anti-TB medication, the predominant bacilli, sensitive to that drug, are killed; the few drug resistant mutants, likely to be present if the bacterial population is large, will multiply freely. Since it is very unlikely that a single bacillus will spontaneously mutate to resistance to more than one drug, giving multiple effective drugs simultaneously will inhibit the multiplication of these resistant mutants.[1]

This book will focus primarily on the people and events surrounding Adirondack Cottage Sanitarium, later to be renamed Trudeau Sanatorium. Edward L. Trudeau, the founder of this sanatorium in Saranac Lake, New York, was known throughout the world as one of the most influential leaders in the nation's campaign against tuberculosis. His sanatorium, the first of its kind in America, became the model for the cure and treatment of TB throughout the United States. Dr. Trudeau's vision and intuition were the guiding forces behind many of the innovative tuberculosis programs that were first pioneered in his sanatorium.

There are many excellent books that describe the history and evolution of the tuberculosis movement in the United States and, more specifically, at Trudeau Sanatorium. Therefore, the focus of this book will primarily be on the human element. It will paint a portrait, through words and pictures, of many of the people who influenced and were influenced by that institution. Although many of the records from the sanatorium have disappeared, every attempt will be made to portray the people and events as accurately as possible.

One of the biggest rewards that came from researching this book was the continuous unearthing of buried treasure: the thoughts, reflections, pictures, letters, and poems of those long gone. Again and again, I was moved to tears, then laughter, then back to tears by what I uncovered. Therefore, much of the text in this book contains, verbatim, those so very eloquently written words that have been hidden for scores of years in dusty archives where few would ever happen upon them. I have attempted to bring some of that glorious prose back to life and, in so doing, create a colorful and, at times, heart rending mosaic portraying those who were healing from tuberculosis at Trudeau Sanatorium.

There was a voice among the mountain's hoar, Crying to those the Great White Fear held fast "Behold, there's hope!"
~Oliver Wilson
Trudeau Memorial Statue Unveiling, 1918

Last Resting Place of Dr. Trudeau

In Their Own Words:
Portrait of Edward Livingston Trudeau

*A*t 11:40 a.m. on a dreary November day, the man, who for forty-three years had refused to die, quietly surrendered to the disease he had spent so long trying to conquer. On November 15, 1915, his long time archenemy, the *tubercle bacillus*, finally claimed Dr. Edward Livingston Trudeau at age sixty-seven. So loved was this gentle man of wisdom, that on the day of his funeral all the stores in the tiny village of Saranac Lake, New York closed; and it was said that "a hush descended upon the entire village."[1]

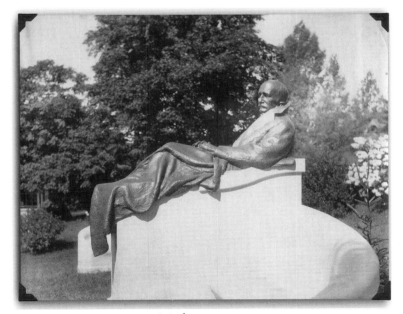

Trudeau Statue
Courtesy of the Trudeau Institute Archives

This was no ordinary victory, this triumph of the "tubercle bacillus." Shorn of its secrets, stripped of much of its mystery, the invisible foe marches on just a little less of a terror to mankind than forty-three years ago when it joined mortal combat with this many-sided man, frail in physique but dominant in personality, with the simplicity of a child, the intuition of a woman, and the sympathy of a man who has felt . . . forty-three years of fight had left their mark. [He was] a long thin man,—long thin feet and legs, a long, thin body, a long, thin face with a long, thin nose and surmounted by a long but massive head, a head that never failed to attract attention . . . long arms gracefully disposed, and wonderfully expressive, long, thin hands adding meaning to all he said to you. . . . His whole attitude was one of interest and eagerness. . . . His crisp, incisive, rapid speech was in harmony with the physical man. . . . The eagerness of Dr. Trudeau's whole bearing indicated at once his intense zest for life. . . . With his right hand he gathered; with his left he gave. And his left hand often moved more swiftly than his right . . . he suffered and enjoyed alike,— intensely . . . he saw and felt his way through life. But with what deftness of touch and what keenness of vision! Dr. Trudeau fitted so gently into his environment and shed his spirit so bountifully over his entire neighborhood that the whole region partook of it and to some extent absorbed Trudeau . . . a brighter and stronger flame [has] lighted the drear Adirondacks.[2]

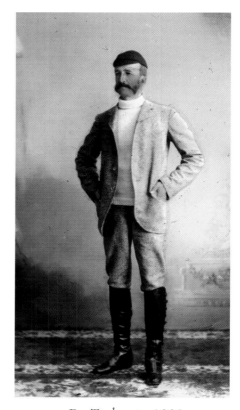

Dr. Trudeau in 1893
Courtesy of the Trudeau Institute Archives

A headline in the local newspaper referred to him as, "A noble citizen who built a town."[3] The Adirondack Cottage Sanitarium, that he founded in 1884, became a haven for those suffering from tuberculosis, and was responsible for bringing hundreds of people and their families to Saranac Lake each year. Thousands of people from around the world owed their lives and health to this kind and giving man. What were the events and circumstances surrounding this noble man of healing that caused an entire world to mourn his passing?

One cannot help but wonder if his heritage predisposed Edward Livingston Trudeau, who was born on October 5, 1848, to choose not only medicine, but also medicine in the wilderness. His mother, Céphise Berger, was the daughter of François Éloi Berger, a French physician who had a prominent practice in New York City, and "whose ancestors were physicians for many generations, as far back as they could be traced."[4] His father, Dr. James de Berty Trudeau, and father-in-law were both founders of the New York Academy of Medicine. His father was also an outdoor enthusiast, and close friend of John J. Audubon, the distinguished naturalist. Audubon named a bird after Trudeau's father who was also credited for several drawings and the anatomy work of Audubon's ornithology. His parents separated soon after his birth and, when Edward was three, he moved to Paris with his mother, brother, and grandparents.

Although Trudeau remembered little about his father, he did know that he had some artistic talent. James Trudeau loved to draw, paint, and had a talent for modeling in clay and casting bronze bas-reliefs. In fact his talent for caricature "had done him an immeasurable amount of harm professionally in New York, for he made a set of statuette caricatures of the medical faculty, which were so well done and such telling caricature that many of the gentlemen never forgave him."[5] These are on permanent display in the Malloch Rare Book Room at the New York Academy of Medicine.

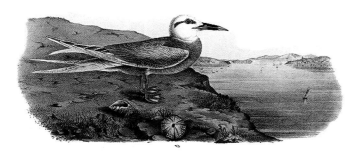

Trudeau's Tern
Courtesy of Haleysteeele.com

According to Trudeau, "The love of wild nature and of hunting was a real passion with my father—a passion which ruined his professional career . . . for he was constantly absent on hunting expeditions."[6] Sometime around 1840, his father and allegedly John Audubon were with John C. Frémont on his expedition to the Rocky Mountains. On his return, an Osage deputy met the expedition and invited Trudeau's father to spend some time with the Osage Indians. The following account, in a letter to Trudeau by his stepmother written after his father's death, details the events that led to that two-year visit:

Your great-grandfather . . . when Governor of 'Les Illinois', in sailing down the Mississippi in his barge from St. Louis to New Orleans, had rescued an Osage chief who had been wounded in a fight on the banks of the river, taken him to his plantation, had him cared for, and when restored to health, helped him to get back to his wigwam and friends. On leaving your parent he had said: 'Indian never forgets;' therefore your father was honored. He always mentioned that his stay with the tribe had been most agreeable and enjoyable, affording him an opportunity to study their customs and manners, learn their language and an ability to ride and use their arms as they did. The costume with which he is represented, was embroidered and presented to him by the squaws of the Osages.[7]

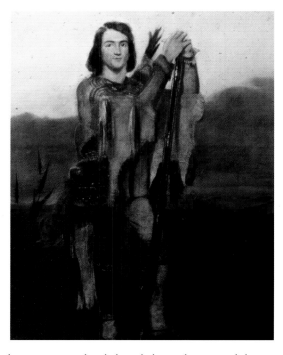

Trudeau's stepmother believed that John J. Audubon painted this oil painting of James Trudeau. John Woodhouse Audubon, his son, was later believed to have been the artist.
Courtesy of the Trudeau Institute Archives

It was this very passion for the wilderness that led young Dr. Trudeau, thought to be dying with consumption in 1872, to "bury [himself] in the Adirondacks—then an unbroken wilderness, and considered a most dangerous climate for a chest invalid—in order to lead an open-air life in the great forest, alone with Nature."[8] Ironically, it was this same "venturesome and pioneer spirit of the Trudeau stock which, turned constructive in the city-bred doctor, blazed new paths and created so much of lasting worth."[9]

Trudeau remained in Paris, attending school where he learned "little in the way of lessons, but a great deal that was bad for me . . . [and how] not to get caught,"[10] until after the war in 1865, when he returned to New York City. He divided his time between New York City in the winters and Nyack on the Hudson in the summers. His life consisted of "joyous play-days . . . horse and wagon . . . sailing . . . and many love affairs."[11]

It was in Nyack, shortly after his return to New York, where young Edward met Lottie Beare, the daughter of an Episcopal minister, who some years later was to become his wife.

Nevertheless it was the tall, slender girl in black, . . who soon inspired me with a love which made me in time give up all the wild mode of life into which I was fast slipping in New York, and work for three years to obtain a medical degree, and for a lifetime to try to be worthy of her. I am often asked if I would be willing to live my life over again, and as I look back on most of it I can say very positively "I have my doubts" but that part which has been lived in contact with the "tall and slender girl. . ." I would gladly live over again indefinitely.[12]

In the fall of 1865, just as Edward was getting ready to enter the Naval Academy, he received word that his older brother, Francis, was ill with tuberculosis. He at once gave up his appointment to the Naval Academy and returned to his grandfather's house in New York to care for his brother. As there were no trained nurses until 1873 when The New England Hospital for Women and Children graduated its first class,[13] Edward assumed total care of his brother for three months, until he died in December of 1865. He tried to cheer him up; he nursed him, and when he could no longer walk, carried him downstairs on his back. During that time, they occupied the same room and often the same bed, and were advised never to open the window, as it would aggravate the cough. At the very end, against medical advice, Edward did open the window because his brother asked for fresh air. The event of his brother's illness and death was a pivotal event in Edward's life and seemed to portend all that was to come.

How strange that, after helping stifle my brother and infect myself through such teaching as was then in vogue, I should have lived to save my own life and that of many others by the simple expedients of an abundance of fresh air. . . . This was my first introduction to tuberculosis and to death. . . . It was my first great sorrow . . . and I have never ceased to feel its influence. In after years it developed in me an unquenchable sympathy for all tuberculosis patients—a sympathy, which I hope, has grown no less through a lifetime spent in trying to express it.[14]

Following the death of his beloved brother, Trudeau found much consolation in the many visits he paid to Lottie Beare's home. He had some measure of company in his sorrow as Lottie's mother and sister had both died two years before the death of Edward's brother.

As time passed, I found that the hours spent in the little cottage by the roadside, inhabited by the saintly clergyman and presided over by his charming daughter, who helped her father with his parish work, played the organ on Sunday, and was beloved by the rich and poor . . . brought more peace to my sorrowing spirit than I could find anywhere else.[15]

After trying a variety of occupations and failing at them all, Trudeau listened to what he termed his "auto-suggestion" and, in 1868, entered medical school at the College of Physicians and Surgeons, the oldest and, perhaps, the best of the three medical schools in New York City. Unbeknown to him at this time, his gift of "auto-suggestion" would soon lead him to create a small city of healing on the side of a mountain that would ultimately change the way the world thought about tuberculosis.

Although Trudeau's friends bet $500 that he would never graduate, he took his studies very seriously. He admitted to feeling very proud of his new *Gray's Anatomy* book and "two venerable human bones" that he was given to study. It took him many grueling hours to determine the anatomical derivation of those bones. This self-teaching of anatomy was his turning point between an easy life and one of work and responsibility.

Medical school teachings were very simple in those days.

There was no entrance examination. All the student had to do was to matriculate at the college and pay a fee of five dollars, attend two or more courses of lectures at the college, and pass the very brief oral examinations which each professor gave the members of the graduating class on his own subject. In addition, the law required that every student enter his name with some reputable practicing physician for three years as a student in his office— a rather hazy and indefinite relation, for which he paid the physician one hundred dollars each year. If these requirements were met the long-hoped-for sheepskin was forthcoming, and the new M.D. was turned loose on the world to meet as best he could the complicated responsibilities of a medical career.[16]

On teaching and lectures at the medical school Trudeau stated:

There was very little clinical or bedside teaching. . . . The teaching was all done by lectures and charts on the wall. . . . The lectures on Medicine and Surgery were didactic. . . . Pathology was taught by the Chair of Medicine as a side issue. No laboratory microscopic studies were required. . . . The theories as to the causation of disease were discussed . . . but the exciting causes of these diseases remained necessarily theoretical.[17]

On tuberculosis, he was taught:

It was a non-contagious, generally incurable and inherited disease, due to inherited constitutional peculiarities, perverted humors and various types of inflammation.[18]

During Trudeau's second winter at medical school, he was feeling fatigued. A doctor examined him and found nothing more than a cold abscess. Although he did not know it at the time, this was his first manifestation of tuberculosis.

Upon graduation from medical school in 1871, he became house physician at the Stranger's Hospital in New York City. Thin and worn out, Trudeau left on June 20, 1871, after his six-month service.

Eight days later he married Lottie Beare. In England, on their honeymoon, he noticed swelling of the lymph glands on his neck. A physician told him the swelling was a result of his run-down condition. Trudeau still did not realize that he was infected with the same disease that had killed his brother.

They returned to New York and Trudeau started a practice on Long Island. Here they rejoiced in the birth of a daughter Charlotte (Chatte) and had a year of happiness and peace. However, that was soon to change. In order to advance his profession, Trudeau decided to move to New York City. Although he had episodic fevers in Long Island, which he attributed to malaria, upon his return to New York City he began to feel constant fatigue. He finally went to be examined at Bellevue Hospital and was told he had tuberculosis.

Upon hearing the diagnosis, Trudeau was devastated and, based on his experience with his brother, he assumed only the worst.

It seemed to me the world had suddenly grown dark. The sun was shining, it is true, and the street was filled with the rush and noise of traffic, but to me the world had lost every vestige of brightness. I had consumption—that most fatal of diseases! Had I not seen it in all its horrors in my brother's case? It meant death and I had never thought of death before! Was I ready to die? How could I tell my wife whom I had just left in unconscious happiness with the little baby in our new home? And my rose-colored dreams of achievement and professional success in New York! They were all shattered now, and in their place only exile and the inevitable end remained! [19]

By the time he reached home, however, Trudeau had already tried to make positive the very ominous news he had just received. Optimism was part of Trudeau's temperament and would later play a significant role in the treatment of his patients at the sanatorium. He was advised to go south, live outdoors, and ride on horseback. Following these orders, he and his wife, again pregnant, left for South Carolina in February 1873. He returned to New York in April with no signs of improvement.

Into the Wilderness (1873 - 1882)

Trudeau thought that he had only a short time to live and, recalling happy memories of time spent hunting in the Adirondacks, he decided to return to the "peace of the wilderness." After a sad parting from his wife, daughter, and one-week-old son Ned, he began his journey into the wilderness on May 25, 1873.

I was influenced in my choice of the Adirondacks only by my love for the great forest and the wild life, and not at all because I thought the climate would be beneficial in any way, for the Adirondacks were then visited only by hunters and fishermen and it was looked upon as a rough, inaccessible region and considered a most inclement and trying climate. I had been to Paul Smith's in the summer on two occasions before . . . and had been greatly attracted by the

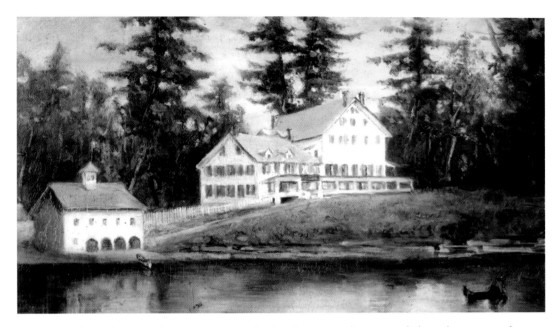

Paul Smith's Hotel on St. Regis Lake. Trudeau's mother painted this oil painting of
Paul Smith's in 1874 during her only visit to the Adirondacks. It now hangs in
Paul Smith's College library on the same site.
Courtesy of the Trudeau Institute Archives

beautiful lakes, the great forest, the hunting and fishing, and the novelty of the free and wild life
there. If I had but a short time to live, I yearned for surroundings that appealed to me.[20]

At that time, Paul Smith, who was a well-known Adirondack guide, ran a primitive hotel on St. Regis Lake a few miles from Saranac Lake. Although drinking water had to be hand carried from a nearby stream, it was a favorite place for "New York's fashionable rich, who liked to listen to Smith's cagily rustic stories, eat his wife's home cooking, and hunt deer and bear in the woods behind his hostelry."[21] It was at Paul Smith's that Trudeau would later meet many of the influential people who would offer financial support for his yet-to-be conceived mission for healing in the wilderness.

After a long and arduous journey by train, boat, and two-horse wagon on which was fashioned a makeshift bed so that he could rest comfortably, Trudeau finally arrived at Paul Smith's. Mrs. Smith's brother carried him up two flights of stairs and on laying him upon his bed remarked:

> *"Why, Doctor, you don't weigh no more than a dried lamb-skin!" We both laughed, and indeed I was so happy at reaching my destination and seeing the beautiful lake again, the mountains and the forest all around me, that I could hardly have been depressed. . . . During the entire journey I had felt gloomy forebodings as to the hopelessness of my case, but under the magic influence of the surroundings I had longed for, these all disappeared and I felt convinced I was going to recover. How little I knew, as I shook hands with the great, strong men who came up to my room that evening to say a word of cheer to me, that forty-two years later most of them would be dead and that I should still be in the Adirondacks and trying to describe my first arrival at Paul Smith's as an invalid! Soon . . . Mrs. Paul Smith's pretty sister, came in with a word of welcome and cheer and a tray on which were eggs, brook trout, pancakes and coffee, and I ate heartily and with a real relish for the first time in many a long week.*[22]

The next morning he spent lying comfortably in a boat that his guide had transformed into a bed with balsam boughs and blankets so that he could recline, his hunting rifle within reach, and enjoy the shimmering reflection of spring green foliage and crisp blue Adirondack sky in the still, clear lake. He felt transformed. His sprits were high, his appetite returned, and he quickly forgot the misery and sense of impending doom that had been weighing him down so heavily less than twenty-four hours before.

> *The change, the stimulus of renewed hope and the constant open-air life had a wonderful effect on my health. I soon began to eat and sleep, and lost my fever. At that time we had no idea of the essential value of rest, but as I often spent the entire day in the boat, fishing or being rowed about from place to place or watching the lake for deer, I unconsciously was kept at rest.*[23]

In Trudeau's mind, he was living proof of the healing effect of the beautiful environs that were the Adirondacks. Ultimately, good food, rest, and open-air therapy became the core components of treatment at the sanatorium.

Even before Trudeau's experience in the woods, William Murray, a pastor from Boston, began vacationing at Racquette Lake in 1866. He believed that the pines emitted large amounts of healing ozone and that the resinous odors from the evergreens had a beneficial effect on the sick. *Adventures in the Wilderness*, which Murray published in 1869, was widely read by those journeying to the Adirondacks. It is not known whether or not Trudeau read this book, which embraced the curative qualities of the Adirondacks.

> *The air which you there inhale is such as can be found only in high mountainous regions, pure, rarefied, and bracing. . . . The spruce, hemlock, balsam, and pine, which largely compose this wilderness, yield upon the air, and especially at night, all their curative qualities. Many a night have I laid down upon my bed of balsam-boughs and been lulled to sleep by the murmur of waters and the low sighing melody of the pines, while the air was laden with the mingled perfume of cedar, of balsam and the water lily.* [24]

Young Dr. Trudeau rejoined his wife at the end of September. He returned a very different man than had entered the wilderness only four months before. He had gained fifteen pounds and believed he had been restored to his previous state of good health. Shortly after returning to New York, however, his old fever returned. He was advised to winter in St. Paul, Minnesota, as the profuse sunshine was thought to have a positive effect on those suffering from pulmonary disease. By spring, he was nearly as sick as he had been the year prior. Once again, in May of 1874, he journeyed back into the Adirondacks, but this time with his wife and two small children. On his return visit to the land he loved he wrote:

> *I have been taken to Paul Smith's from Saranac Lake in the spring so ill that my life was despaired of; and yet little by little, while lying out under the great trees, looking out on the lake all day, my fever has stopped and my strength slowly begun to return. . . . The magic spell of the old place, however, seemed again able to restore the failing spark of existence.* [25]

During the summer of 1874, however, Trudeau did not improve as markedly as he had the previous summer. Tired of traveling back and forth from New York City, he proposed to Dr. Alfred Loomis, a recovered consumptive and new friend that he had met while at Paul Smith's, the idea of remaining in the Adirondacks for the winter. Loomis believed that Trudeau would probably die before winter's end and, therefore, could see no reason he shouldn't spend his remaining days in a place that brought him such happiness. In fact, Loomis advised another of his patients to remain for the winter as well.

Wintering in the Adirondacks required overcoming numerous obstacles. First, he had to convince his wife. They would be cut off from all connections to the outside world. The nearest doctor was at Plattsburgh; a sixty-mile horse-carriage drive away over often poorly defined roads. Mail arrived three times a week at neighboring Bloomingdale, a ten-mile drive away.

> *My wife, however, has never been the nervous, overanxious type, but always self-contained, meeting quietly and bravely all the ills and sorrows that have come to us in life. We were young and happy together with our children, and were not inclined to borrow trouble; thus it came about that we decided to face the terrors of an Adirondack winter.*[26]

He then had to convince Mrs. Smith, as no "outsider" had ever spent a winter at St. Regis Lake before.

> *The truth, I imagine, was that Mrs. Smith feared I never would live through the winter, and I know they both thought it a most rash and foolish thing for such a sick man to do. In those days the belief that cold and storm were the two things to be avoided by the consumptive, and that he should in winter seek a warm and sunny climate, was so general and deep-rooted that my staying in so rough a climate seemed to them little short of suicide.*[27]

In the middle of January 1875, Edward drove forty miles from Paul Smith's to Malone in a small horse drawn cutter to meet his little family who were joining him from New York City. Their return trip took more than forty-eight hours. Paul Smith later commented about the long trip home:

> *I went down with two big heavy teams—he had a lot of stuff to come up—and the doctor took his horse and cutter. We got to Malone and I guess we stayed there one day. It snowed all the time. But we loaded up the next day and started for home. Got to Duane, fourteen miles, and*

we were in the snow all day long; the horses up to their sides in the snow. I took the children out, cut a hole in the snow, put a blanket in . . . and put them in this big snow hole, and there they stayed until we got the horses through the drifts.[28]

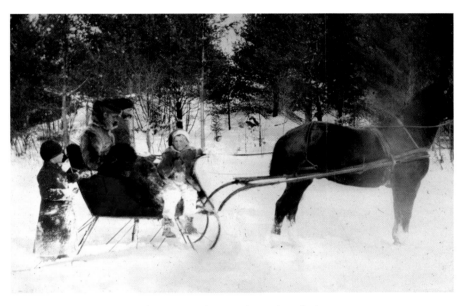

Dr. and Mrs. Trudeau with Ned and playmate
Courtesy of the Trudeau Institute Archives

During their first winter when the snow reached a depth of five feet in the woods, Trudeau did well, rarely had any fever, and, in spite of his rough surroundings, had a happy winter with his family.

In the summer, when the guests returned, they were surprised that Trudeau had survived an Adirondack winter in the wilderness. Up until that time, he was so intent on his own survival that he had nearly forgotten that he was a physician. But as the summer guests occasionally needed medical attention, he slowly began to practice medicine in the woods. He remained at Paul Smith's throughout the summer. Though his fever returned, his condition had not worsened and so he decided to stay another winter.

As they were unable to stay at Paul Smith's that winter, Trudeau rented a small house in Saranac Lake.

Life in Saranac Lake was simple in those days. There was no coal, no water pipes, and no other light than that which was furnished by kerosene lamp or candle. There were no stores, no churches, and nothing came from the outside world, except when brought by the two horse sleigh which ran daily to Ausable Forks when the roads were passable.[29]

In November 1876, his little family again joined him in the Adirondacks where they would spend their remaining years. He would pass his time during those long winter days by hunting and ultimately begin what was to be his final life-transforming journey into a daring new world.

I never lost my keen interest in hunting, and it has remained an ever-enduring pleasure and relaxation of which I did not allow my physical infirmities to deprive me.[30]

It was during his winters of hunting that he made an important discovery.

I found, however, I could not walk enough to stand much chance for a shot without feeling sick and feverish the next day, and this was the first intimation I had as to the value of the rest cure, which in after years I applied so thoroughly and rigidly to my patients. I walked very little after this, and my faith in the value of the rest cure became more and more fully established.[31]

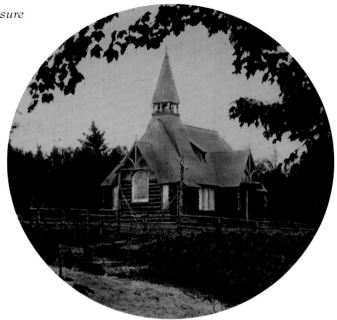

St. John's in the Wilderness
Courtesy of the Trudeau Institute Archives

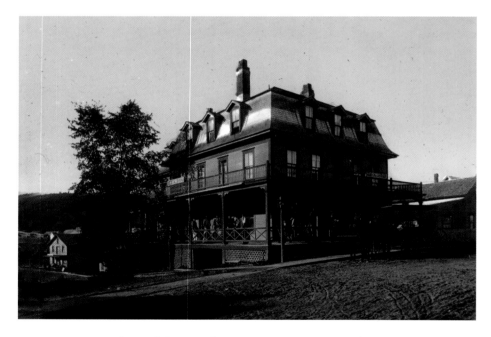

The Berkeley Hotel, Main Street, Saranac Lake
Courtesy of the Trudeau Institute Archives

During the latter part of 1876, Trudeau started collecting money for a little log chapel that was to be built near Paul Smith's. He soon raised enough money to build St. John's in the Wilderness, a little Episcopal chapel, known "far and wide for the originality of its construction and the beauty and simplicity of its design." Every Sunday, in preparation for the church service, his wife adorned the altar with flowers or autumn leaves gathered from the woods that surrounded the little church. Although Trudeau claimed that his primary reason for building the

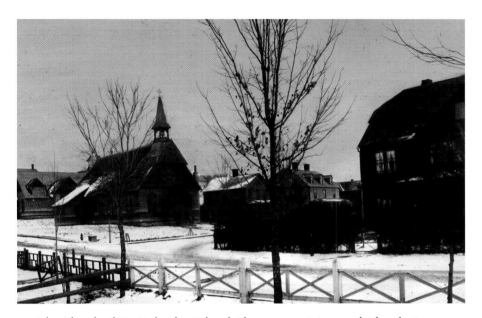

The Church of St. Luke the Beloved Physician on Main and Church Streets
Courtesy of the Trudeau Institute Archives

little church was for the guides' families, one cannot help but wonder if the real reason was to give something of meaning back to his devoted wife, the daughter of an Episcopal minister, who had so uncomplainingly given up her life of comfort in order to care for her sick husband in the wilderness.

In May of 1877, Dr. and Mrs. Trudeau celebrated the birth of their third child, Henry. The following winter Henry had convulsions and died two days later. It was the first of many sorrows that Trudeau and his wife would experience together. Henry was buried beneath the tall pines near the eaves of the little church that his father had so recently built.

As a result of Trudeau's positive healing experiences in Saranac Lake, Dr. Loomis was now recommending that many of his consumptive patients consider wintering there as well. In order to accommodate the increasing numbers of people coming to Saranac Lake, the Berkeley Hotel, with a maximum capacity of twenty guests, was built on Main Street. During the winter months, Episcopal services were held in the parlor of the hotel for visitors as well as residents of Saranac Lake. Therefore, it wasn't long before the residents decided to raise money to build an Episcopal church, later to be named The Church of St. Luke the Beloved Physician. And *who* better equipped to take on the project than Trudeau. In 1878, when asked if he would undertake the building of the church, he replied:

> *I told them I would do as they requested under one condition, namely, that I was to have entire charge, and that I was to be allowed to build the church steeple downward and the foundation upward if I saw fit. This they agreed to. When I told my wife of this she smiled, and said she had often noticed that I was fond of having my own way. My own way seemed to answer the*

purpose . . . the church was built without the slightest friction. . . . Work was begun May, 1878, and the church was finished January, 1879.[32]

Although he had built two churches, Trudeau claimed that, until the early 1880s, he did little but hunt and fish.

But loving the woods he found solace in the aroma of the pines, the soothing melody of the rippling brooks, and the forest life. To him as a woodsman the forest was a constantly varying source of joy, not only in the present, but in anticipation and in reminiscence. The pulsating drum of the strutting grouse, the widening swirl of the feeding trout, or it may be a deer with outstretched neck and flaring ears stepping warily out upon the marsh, awakened memories which became reveries in the semi-somnolent comfort round the camp fire, as it cast its enfolding warmth. And so the early days of convalescence passed in quiet contentment, bringing increasing vigor and permitting a renewal of the hunting trips which afforded him such recreation and enjoyment. It was upon one of these trips that he conceived the Adirondack Cottage Sanitarium project and decided upon its site.[33]

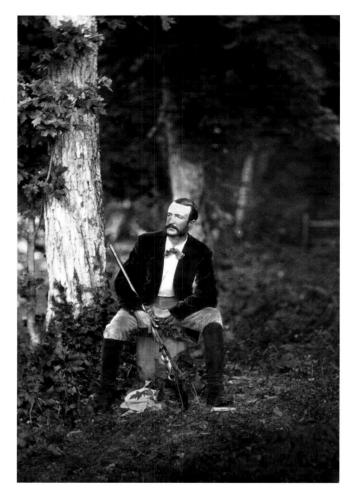

Dr. Trudeau, the Huntsman, three months after his arrival at Paul Smith's in 1873
Courtesy of the Trudeau Institute Archives

In 1882 Trudeau learned of two events happening in Europe that would have a ripple effect from across the ocean directly into Saranac Lake. While reading his medical journals, Trudeau first learned of Hermann Brehmer's Tuberculosis Sanitarium in Silesia and also of Robert Koch's work on the identification of the *tubercle bacillus.*

> *Brehmer was the originator of the sanatorium method, the essence of which was rest, fresh air and a daily regulation by the physician of the patient's life and habits. Brehmer, however, had an idea that tuberculosis of the lungs was somewhat dependent on, or at least related to, a small heart, and after the fever had fallen he attached much importance to graded climbing exercises for his patients to strengthen the heart.*
>
> *Dettweiler, a patient and pupil of his, built a sanatorium at Falkenstein in Germany, here he followed Brehmer's method, except that Dettweiler was an ardent advocate of complete rest, and he did not believe that a small heart had any special relation to pulmonary tuberculosis.*
>
> *I was much impressed with the articles I read on the subject in the "English Practitioner," and though I saw no reference to either Brehmer's or Dettweiler's work in my American journals, I became desirous of making a test of this new method in treating some of my tuberculosis patients.*[34]

An idea had been born! Trudeau's gift of "auto-suggestion" once more was feeding his bright and creative mind with a revolutionary way he could provide a healing environment to the many invalids, stricken with tuberculosis, who had nowhere to turn for help.

> *I was also much impressed at that time with the difficulty of obtaining suitable accommodations in the Adirondacks for patients of moderate means. The rich and well-to-do could hire one of the few guides' cottages in Saranac Lake or pay them well for taking them to board, but there was absolutely no place for the working men and women who came here with short purses. It therefore occurred to me that a good piece of work could be done in helping these invalids, for whom my*

sympathy ever since my brother's death had always been keen, by building a few small cottages where they could be taken at a little less than cost, and where the sanatorium method could be tried.[35]

From the onset, Trudeau planned to charge nothing for his services. However, he needed to raise money from his wealthy patients and many friends for the small cottages and land on which the sanatorium would be built. He also had to determine the best location. None of these tasks remained obstacles for long.

Trudeau believed that the location of his sanatorium should provide the same type of environment that was so healing to him years before when, for the first time, he had come to die. So Trudeau went to his favorite fox runway, where he had spent so many happy days, and there he found the perfect spot. How much it says about the extreme selflessness of this man that, in the name of healing, he would give up the very same piece of land that had brought so much joy and comfort to him throughout the years.

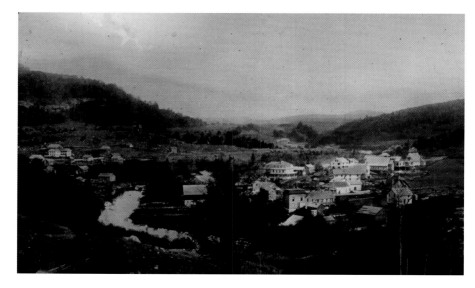

Saranac Lake Vista. In the upper left, nestled on the side of the mountain, can be seen the location of the sanatorium. The Village of Saranac Lake is in the foreground.
Courtesy of the Trudeau Institute Archives

Here the mountains, covered with an unbroken forest, rose so abruptly from the river, and the sweep of the valley at their base was so extended and picturesque, that the view had always made a deep impression upon me. Many a beautiful afternoon, for the first four winters after I came to Saranac Lake, I had sat for hours alone while hunting, facing the ever-changing phases of light and shade on the imposing mountain panorama at my feet, and dreamed the dreams of youth; dreamed of life and death and God, and yearned for a closer contact with the Great Spirit who planned it all, and for light on the hidden meaning of our troublous existence. The grandeur and peace of it had ever brought refreshment to my perplexed spirit.[36]

Fitz Greene Hallock was not only an Adirondack guide; he was also one of Trudeau's most loyal friends. Fitz spread the word among the other guides from Paul Smith's about the piece of land that Trudeau was interested in purchasing for his sanatorium. Much to Trudeau's surprise and delight, the guides presented him with the deed for the land after they had chipped in and bought the sixteen acres for twenty-five dollars an acre. The guides were a very important part of Adirondack lore.

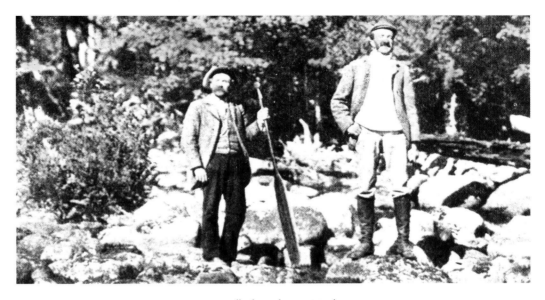

Fitz Hallock with Dr. Trudeau
Courtesy of the Trudeau Institute Archives

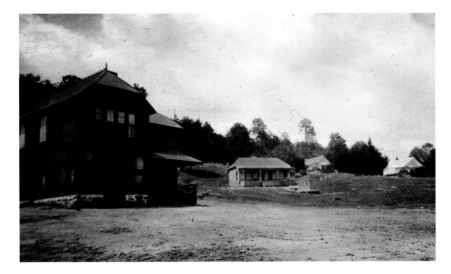

The Adirondack Cottage Sanitarium in 1885
Courtesy of the Trudeau Institute Archives

The old Adirondack guides were most striking personalities and an interesting lot of men . . . a happy, easy-going lot, who took no care for the morrow and enjoyed life for life's sake . . . each guide had his specialty . . . really good guides were certainly experts at their business, and easily earned their two and a half or three dollars a day. A good guide was first of all a truthful man whose work could be relied upon; he was a skilled oarsman, and often carried his boat on his back for miles from one lake to another; a thorough woodsman, with all that implies of fishing, hunting and wood-lore; a good cook, resourceful in emergencies, and an excellent companion.[37]

The money for Trudeau's new venture began coming in. After one trip to New York City in 1883, he collected over $3,000. One woman from Boston sent him a check for $25,000. When Trudeau received that check he claimed that he rubbed his eyes in disbelief because it seemed to contain way too many "ciphers." He was ready to construct his first building at the Adirondack Cottage Sanitarium, the first of its kind in this country. Trudeau admitted that he had no knowledge of what type of buildings he should plan nor was that information available to him in books. Intuitively, he believed that patients would be better off housed in small cottages rather than grouped together in large wards.

> By adopting this plan an abundant supply of air could be secured for the patient, the irritation of constant close contact with many strangers could be avoided, and I knew it would be easier to get some of my patients to give a little cottage which would be their own individual gift, rather than a corresponding sum of money toward the erection of larger buildings. . . . When later the transmissibility of tuberculosis . . . became generally accepted, I had reason to be thankful that I had from the first adopted the cottage plan.[38]

During the fall of 1884, his first two patients arrived and were housed in part of the nearly completed main building that consisted of a little sitting room, a dining room, kitchen, and accommodations for the administration department. The following year "The Little Red," the first cottage, was completed. Little Red consisted of:

> one room, fourteen by eighteen, and a little porch so small that only one patient could sit out at a time, and with difficulty. It was furnished with a wood stove, two cot-beds, a washstand, two chairs and a kerosene lamp, and cost, as I remember, about four hundred dollars when completed.[39]

Trudeau's credo—"to cure sometimes, to relieve often, to comfort always"—and his philosophy of healing, which included air, rest, food, and positive attitude, began to spread. Remembering his experience in caring for his brother as well as the healing effect of the environment on

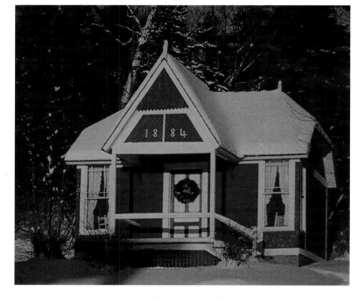

The Little Red
Courtesy of the Trudeau Institute Archives

his own illness, he was determined that he would provide care for the whole person, not just the physical component. His approach would emphasize the spiritual, psychological, social, and biological aspects of care.

What was it like to be a patient in Little Red? Carolyn Lindsay tells of her experience at Little Red in 1887. She left New York with her sister on a mild February day. En route, they encountered a "narrow canon of snow" and were to have been met at the railroad in Loon Lake with fur coats which never materialized. They arrived at the main building of the sanatorium during the worst blizzard in seventeen years.

Things were not altogether ideal then in the early development of what was afterwards a huge enterprise. The water system was not adequate; sputum cups . . . were not used. But our daily ride in winter, wrapped in fur coats, and with hot bricks at our feet, was almost a dissipation; and the arrival of the stage with the mail and a possible express package was excitement enough to cause a run of fever. . . . We indulged in splitting birch bark, gathering spruce gum, and in the spring gathering the most beautiful mountain violets, picking wild strawberries and later marvelous blueberries.

The long, boot-covered legs with the purposeful stride that were Dr. Trudeau's were an inspiration to a discouraged patient . . . he radiated happiness in the very way he would throw off that sealskin cap and laugh. . . . Commenting upon a patient's singing one day, he said her voice was "hollow" but "no wonder, for she had a hole in her left lung you could put your fist in." He encouraged singing and whistling as helpful agencies. . . . His prescriptions were few, for he depended upon air, food and rest for the cure.

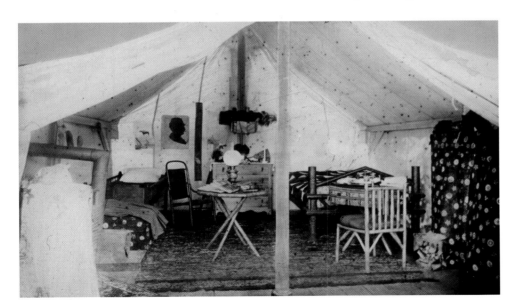

Cure Tents, donated in 1884, were part of the Cottage Plan
Courtesy of the Trudeau Institute Archives

Numerous "cures" were tried out by Dr. Trudeau. One was a sulphide of hydrogen gas treatment that smelled like decayed eggs. Another was breathing a medicated oxygen as the victim sat shut up in a glass cabinet for a stated period daily.

The board rate was $5.00 a week. There were accommodations for about twenty-five patients when the few cottages were full. . . . Little by little the gospel of air, rest, and food for tuberculosis spread. The patients were the only advertisers in those days. We who were benefited in those early days are glad to say "thank you and God bless Doctor Trudeau" and if the writer has done any real good in the world, much of the credit is due to that wonderful year of life at the Sanatorium where my dear sister, Annie, and I lived so happily in the "Little Red" cottage.[40]

Hermann Brehmer's and Peter Dettweiler's methods for the sanatorium treatment of tuberculosis patients served to confirm what experience had already taught Trudeau. His own life's lessons during his first journey into the wilds nearly ten years before had, in his mind, dramatically demonstrated the positive effects of an abundance of fresh pine-filled air, wholesome food, regulated rest, and plenty of nonstrenuous activities that promoted feelings of happiness, usefulness, and extreme satisfaction. A second major discovery confirmed another theory that he had also begun to believe in.

Koch published a paper in Germany in 1882, which described the identification of the bacterium—the *tubercle bacillus*—which was responsible for causing tuberculosis.

There was every reason why this announcement of Koch's should make a deep impression on me. I was already familiar with Tyndall's and Pasteur's work on the origin of life, and Pasteur had only recently asserted . . . that putrefaction was caused by living germs, which could be cultivated and studied at will. . . . Lister found that if wounds could be kept free from contamination by germs by the use of carbolic acid they would heal without any suppuration. I also had read a statement of Pasteur's belief that all infectious diseases came from living germs.

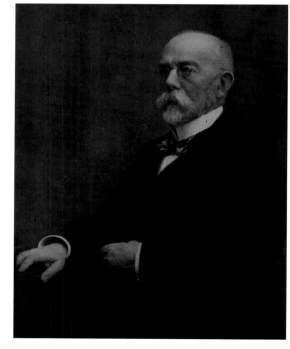

Robert Koch
Courtesy of the Trudeau Institute Archives

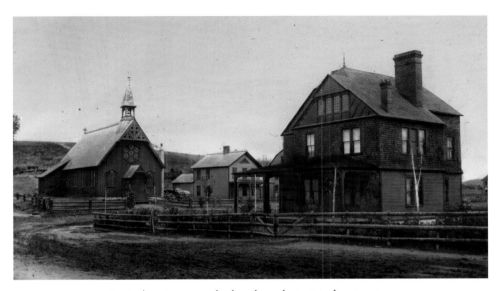

St. Luke's Episcopal Church and Dr. Trudeau's Home
Courtesy of the Trudeau Institute Archives

This time in medicine was the dawn of the achievements of the new experimental method —a method which was casting so much light on dark places—and the glamor of its possibilities in the prevention and cure of disease took a strong hold on my imagination.[41]

Even though other physicians in the country were not convinced of the value of Koch's discovery, Trudeau immediately wanted to duplicate his work. On his next visit to New York City, Trudeau spent the entire time learning how to stain and recognize the *tubercle bacillus*. He returned home and, in the fall of 1885, immediately began to equip his recently constructed Queen Anne cottage, located near St. Luke's Episcopal Church, with a small (twelve by eight feet) laboratory. This was the first laboratory in the world devoted exclusively to the study of tuberculosis. After he perfected staining and recognizing the bacillus, he learned how to culture it outside the body so he could begin to produce the disease in animals for the purpose of experimentation. He became the first person in the United States to isolate the bacteria.

Back in Saranac Lake a room in the little frame cottage soon became a laboratory, with equipment for the most part home-made and painfully fashioned by a lone exile, who meanwhile went through zero and the snows to see his patients. And there, for years by himself, he taught himself his own techniques, applied this to the study of tuberculosis, and made discoveries.[42]

Now that he had been able to isolate the bacteria, he wanted to determine whether or not rest, fresh air, and food really did make a difference once the germ had been introduced into the body. In 1887 Trudeau published the results of the following study which gave much acclaimed scientific evidence of the interaction between environment and disease.

Lot 1, of five rabbits, were inoculated with pure cultures and put under the best surrounding of light, food, and air attainable. [These] were turned loose on a little island in front of my camp at Paul Smith's, where they ran wild all summer in the fresh air and sunshine, and were provided abundant food.

Lot 2, of five rabbits, inoculated at the same time and in the same way, were put under the worst conditions of environment I could devise. [These] were put in a dark, damp place where the air was bad, confined in a small box and fed insufficiently.

Lot 3, of five rabbits, were put under similar bad conditions without being inoculated. [These were also] put in a dark, damp place where the air was bad, confined in a small box and fed insufficiently.

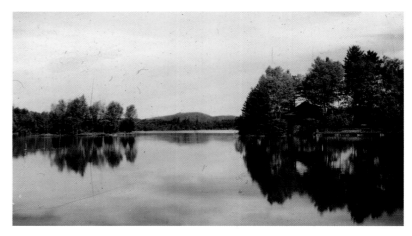

Rabbit Island, on the left, where Trudeau conducted his experiment
Courtesy of the Trudeau Institute Archives

The results showed that of the rabbits allowed to run wild under good conditions, all, with one exception, recovered. Of lot 2, . . four rabbits died within three months and the organs showed extensive tuberculosis. Lot 3, uninoculated animals, . . though emaciated, they showed no signs of the disease.[43]

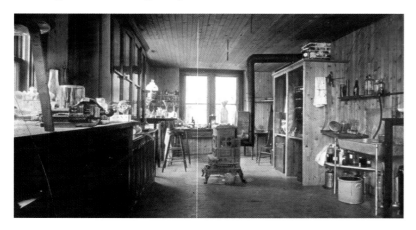

Interior of Dr. Trudeau's first home laboratory
Courtesy of the Trudeau Institute Archives

In Trudeau's mind, this lent strong support to the treatment protocol that he was using in his fledgling sanatorium. It also encouraged him to continue seeking financial backing in order to expand the sanatorium. By 1887 the Main Building had been finished and enlarged, and four other cottages had been constructed.

But all was not easy. There was still no running water or coal, and he was constantly plagued by an inadequate drainage system. In the summers, when he lived at Paul Smith's, he had to make the twice a week round trip commute of twenty-eight miles to do the medical work for his patients as he could not afford a doctor in residence at the sanatorium. Furthermore:

I had no nurse nor anyone to direct the patients and encourage them. When they were taken acutely ill with complications I had no infirmary to send them to, and no one to carry their meals and nurse them in their cottages. I used to hire lumberman and guides to care for the bed-ridden men patients, and any old woman I could get to look after the women, and they were very expensive and not very efficient help. In cases of severe hemorrhage these improvised nurses would become panic-stricken and escape from the sick-room, and often no amount of eloquence on my part would induce them to return. On the rare occasions when anybody died I had to come over and take charge of the situation in person, as the entire establishment was thrown into such a panic that I feared they would all desert in a body.[44]

As the years went by, the sanatorium continued to grow in many ways. Numerous buildings were constructed, new staff were hired, better equipment was purchased, and the the fame of Saranac Lake as a health resort began to spread throughout the world. The far reaching reputation of the Adirondack Cottage Sanitarium began to change the way the world viewed consumption.

Dr. Hermann M. Biggs, New York State Commissioner of Health, had the following words of praise for Trudeau's ever increasing influence on the world views of tuberculosis:

Previously, patients suffering with this disease had been most carefully shielded from every breath of fresh air, had been housed in artificially heated rooms, kept at a high and uniform temperature, covered with blankets, fed on liquid food, and drugged with remedies intended to allay the ever harassing

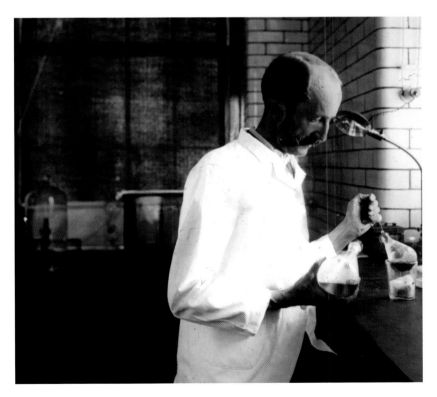

Dr. Trudeau in his new laboratory built in 1894
Courtesy of the Trudeau Institute Archives

cough and to prevent the recurring profuse perspirations and the fever. . . . Instead of the pale, rapidly emaciating sufferer with hectic flush, harassing cough and profuse expectoration, sleepless nights with drenching sweats and an ever increasing intolerance and repugnance to food, [one] sees well nourished patients with tanned cheeks, hearty appetites, almost, or entirely, free from cough, expectoration and fever, daily gaining in weight and strength. For this fundamental change in the method of treatment of pulmonary tuberculosis and in the results obtained, with all that it involves, directly and indirectly; for the change in the outlook in many cases from despair to a hopeful confidence, for the establishment of hundreds of clinics and sanatoria throughout this country; for the approaching universal adoption of the open air method of treatment for the sick, Trudeau's work is responsible to a greater extent than that of any other man or than that of any group of men in this country.[45]

The sanatorium became essentially an experiment in the rehabilitation of the middle-class consumptive. It could pick and choose its patients, and its two prime standards of admission were curability of disease and financial resources that could not meet the average cost of boarding-house residence in Saranac Lake.[46]

Trudeau admitted that his admission requirements often subjected him to criticism by some physicians who believed that he was limiting admissions to only favorable cases for the primary purpose of positively skewing his statistical outcomes. Trudeau, however, realized that early diagnosis was the key to successful treatment and, as he was interested in obtaining curative results, he felt obligated to confine his admissions to incipient and favorable cases only. In response to the critisism he stated, "I have learned, however, that unjust criticism is inevitable in this world, and must be borne calmly so long as one's conscience is clear."[47]

Over the next several years, Trudeau's life would undergo many changes.

*Pleasure and pain
Have followed each other
Like sunshine and rain.*[48]

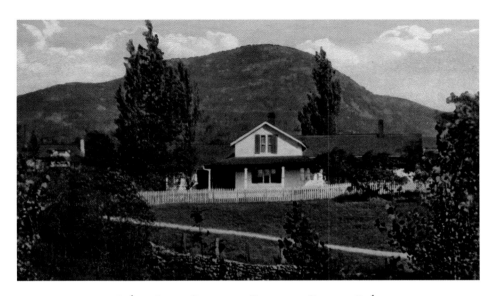

Robert Louis Stevenson Cottage in Saranac Lake
From the postcard collection of Florence H. Wright

*I was walking in the verandah of a small cottage
outside the hamlet of Saranac.
It was winter, the night was very dark, the air
clear and cold, and sweet with the
purity of the forests. For the making of a story
here were fine conditions.
'Come' I said I to my engine,
'let us make a tale'*

~Robert Louis Stevenson

On October 3, 1887, Robert Louis Stevenson arrived in Saranac Lake for his health. He had intended to go to Colorado, but as he wasn't judged strong enough to make the journey he went to Saranac Lake instead. Although Stevenson was Trudeau's patient, he spent the fall and winter in Andrew Baker's cottage on the outskirts of the village rather than at the sanatorium as he was considered financially too well off to be allowed entry at the sanatorium. Trudeau also believed that Stevenson had bronchitis rather than tuberculosis, another factor that most likely impeded his entry. Stevenson referred to his little cottage as "a house in the eye of many winds with a view of a piece of running water."[49]

Although Stevenson intensely disliked the climate, he came to love his little cottage and the surrounding country. Of the climate Stevenson wrote:

*A bleak blackguard beggarly climate, of which I can say no good except that it suits me. . . .
The grayness of the heavens here is a circumstance eminently revolting to the soul.*[50]

Trudeau and Stevenson developed a warm respect for one another during the months that he was in residence. Trudeau related the following story to a group of physicians in Baltimore:

Stevenson naturally looked with repugnance on the exact and uncompromising methods of scientific research and animal experimentation, and we had many heated arguments on this subject. I finally persuaded him one day to visit the little room in my cottage, which was then my only laboratory. He had just written for Scribner's a short essay entitled "The Lantern-Bearers" in which some of his beautiful thoughts had as a text a game he and the other boys played, and which consisted of walking along on a dark night hiding under their coats a lantern which was only flashed at each other as they passed as a signal.

I was intent on showing him my animals and culture tubes, and the ravages which are caused by the "tubercle bacillus" in the organs of animals, and was trying to impress upon him the possibilities which lay in these experiments in advancing our knowledge of a germ which kills one in seven of the human race, when suddenly I noticed that he looked pale, was not listening, and was edging toward the door as fast as possible.

As soon as we got outside he turned to me and said: "Trudeau, your lantern may be very bright to you but to me it smells of oil like the devil!" It was evident that neither of us could appreciate the brightness of each other's lantern, though we both tried.[51]

While Stevenson was at Saranac Lake, he wrote some of his best work: *Pulvis et Umbra*, *The Lantern Bearers*, *A Christmas Sermon*, and parts of *The Master of Ballantrae*. When he wasn't writing, he could often be found skating on Moody Pond or dreaming of warm and distant climates. A scar left by his cigarette burn still adorns the mantle in the little Stevenson Cottage that now bears his name and has become a favorite regional tourist stop.

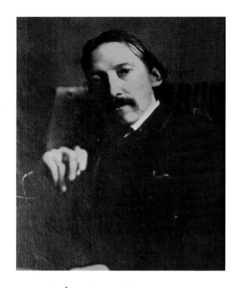

Robert Louis Stevenson at Saranac Lake, 1887-1888
Courtesy of the Trudeau Institute Archives

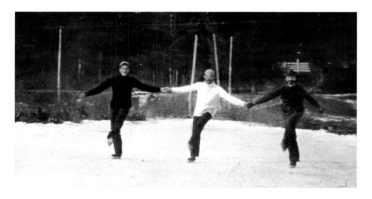

This picture is thought to be of Robert Louis Stevenson (on right) and Dr. Trudeau (center) skating on Moody Pond
Courtesy of the Trudeau Institute Archives

Upon his departure from Saranac Lake, he presented Trudeau with a bound set of his works. Each volume contained a handwritten verse dedicated specifically to each member of the family, including the dog, Nig! Trudeau considered these to be invaluable gifts and treasured them dearly.

It is not hard to imagine whom Stevenson was thinking of when he wrote the following in *Beggars*:

> *You should have heard him speak of what he loved; of the tent pitched beside the talking water; of the peep of day over the moors; the awakening birds among the birches; how he abhorred the long winter-shut-in cities; and with what delight at the return of the spring, he once more pitched his camp in the living out-of-doors.*

Much to the surprise of Dr. and Mrs. Trudeau, a baby boy, Francis, was born in 1887, twelve years after the birth of Ned. Trudeau admitted that:

> *The prospect of bringing up another baby was not very alluring. . . . But Providence plays strange tricks: and it is not always given to us to perceive in today's trial the comfort of tomorrow. . . . The arrival of the new baby was a Godsend to us before many years, as sickness, sorrow and death were soon to cast their dark shadow on our household.*[52]

The same fall that baby Francis was born, Dr. and Mrs. Trudeau decided to send their sixteen-year-old daughter Chatte off to school in New York City so that she could have exposure to greater educational opportunities than were present in little Saranac Lake. Chatte was a strong, vigorous, and athletic girl who loved the outdoors. But during her first semester at school, she was homesick and not very happy in her new surroundings. In January she wrote that she didn't feel well, had lost her appetite, and complained of indigestion. At first Trudeau thought it might be the influence of city life but when her complaints did not abate, he suggested she come home for Easter so that he could examine her. In his autobiography, Trudeau recounts the heartbreaking discovery of the cause of her complaints:

> *I never shall forget the shock her appearance gave me. From a plump, robust young woman she had changed to a pale, listless girl, and as she went upstairs to see her mother I went into my office and shut the door. The terrible truth flashed upon me as I remembered how my brother*

appeared when he was taken ill . . . I knew it was the same old story, and I felt stunned and had to wait a long time to get hold of myself again before joining the family circle. I at once made up my mind I must know the truth, and alarm her as little as possible. It was my responsibility and I could share it with no one, so I did a piece of acting that day which I shall never forget.[53]

Trudeau could not bring himself to write about what really happened the evening of his daughter's homecoming. As the family sat down to the evening meal, he went up to Chatte's room in search of her handkerchief. After finding it, he stole quietly into his laboratory and made a smear of her sputum from the sample in her handkerchief. He found evidence of what he so feared—the *tubercle bacilli*. For many long months, he carried this secret in his saddened heart, sharing it only with his wife who always seemed to be able stand tall under the swift blow of devastating news.[54] With heartbreaking eloquence, Trudeau writes of his daughter's nearly three years of suffering. Here was a man whose life mission had become curing those suffering from tuberculosis. But as Chatte was stricken with the same rapidly progressive type of disease that his brother had died from, this great man of healing could do no more than watch helplessly as his young daughter faded painfully into death.

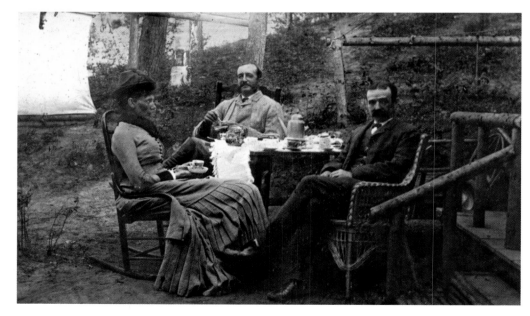

During those sad years of Chatte's struggle for life my wife and I ever lived with heavy hearts, though we tried to show her only smiling faces . . . I had to keep the work at the Sanitarium and Laboratory going, and to that extent I could forget. But for my wife it was much harder, for she was almost always with Chatte, always trying to guide her in her daily life, amusing her, reading to her, trying to make her forget; and I was lost in wonder and admiration as I watched

The Trudeaus entertaining Dr. Luis P. Walton at their camp on Spitfire Lake
Courtesy of the Trudeau Institute Archives

her through these long, trying years, always serene, helpful and cheerful, though I often knew that her heart was breaking. . . . The last winter of Chatte's life she suffered so constantly that it was a terrible strain to us all. As I worked in the little laboratory I could always hear her constant and harassing cough. . . . She died on the night of March 20, 1893, and after she had gone my wife and I, though stunned by the blow we had been expecting for so long, could not but be thankful that her suffering was at an end. . . . We decided to have the funeral at St. Luke's and lay Chatte in the little churchyard at St. Regis by the side of the baby, who was sleeping there under a little white cross. . . . We started for St. Regis in sleighs as soon as the ceremony was over. The snow was four feet deep on the level and drifted in many places. Six strong men had to walk by the coffin and steady it when drifts were encountered by the struggling horses. As we neared St. Regis I could not but go back in memory to the trying trip through the snow from Malone in January, 1875, when Chatte was brought . . . to St. Regis; and she was now being carried in her coffin through the same deep drifts, to the same place, to sleep the "long sleep" by the little church where she had worshipped all through her innocent young life. . . . I felt she would rest more peacefully under the tall pines than anywhere else, and a great peace seemed to come to me with the thought that "all is well with the child." My wife and I sat silently as we drove home through the darkness and the deep snow, and I derived some comfort from repeating to myself these words: "What I do thou knowest not now, but thou shalt know hereafter."[55]

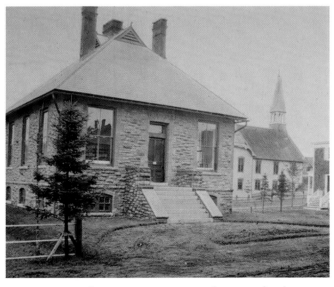

Dr. Trudeau's new Saranac Laboratory for the Study of Tuberculosis. The Methodist church is in the background and his new home is on the right.
Courtesy of the Trudeau Institute Archives

The year of 1893 had not yet finished wielding its harsh blows to Dr. Trudeau. In December of 1893, when he was lying very ill with a kidney abscess in a New York City hotel, he received news that his house and little laboratory had burned to the ground. His precious pen-written translation of Koch's works was destroyed in the fire. The much loved and personally inscribed volumes of Stevenson's writings were also burned to ashes. Within hours his friends and colleagues rallied around his bedside. His friend Mr. George Cooper offered to pay for the construction of a new "stone and steel laboratory; one that will never burn up," and his colleagues from the laboratory in New York, where he had so laboriously learned to stain and recognize the bacilli, presented him with a new microscope. Enclosed with the microscope was the following note:

My dear Doctor Trudeau:

We men at the laboratory want to make you a Christmas present and we are so eager in wanting to that we cannot wait till the proper time. I don't think we have decided whether we want to do this most because we appreciate the good work you are always doing, in our line and others, or because you have more pluck than anybody we know, or because you have been so often helpful to us and made us always glad to have you here, or because—well, the fact is, old fellow, we like you and want you to know it and so here we are in a row, bowing our early Christmas greeting.[50]

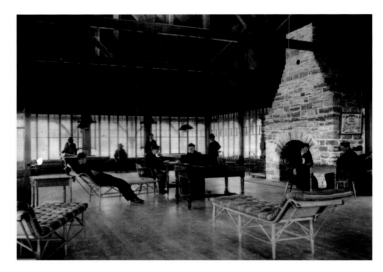

Patients enjoying recreational activities in the Open-Air Pavilion
Courtesy of the Trudeau Institute Archives

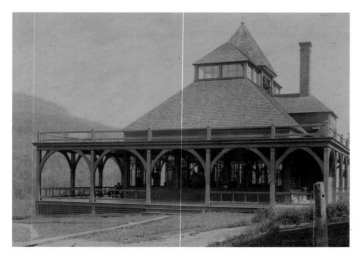

Exterior of Open-Air Pavilion
Courtesy of the Trudeau Institute Archives

Despite the years of sadness, the sanatorium continued to flourish and grow. Nine new cottages were built between 1888 and 1894. An open-air pavilion for recreation was constructed, as was a cottage for the resident physician who was now in attendance. There were a number of physicians who came to the sanatorium to cure, but later remained on to help provide medical care. Dr. Edward Baldwin was one of those physicians. He showed up on Dr. Trudeau's doorstep in 1892, seeking admission to the sanatorium, and stayed on to become Dr. Trudeau's close friend and ultimately director of the laboratory.

A small infirmary cottage for the very ill was also completed. It was at this point that Dr. Trudeau hired Miss Ruth Collins, his first registered nurse, who became a vital and much loved part of the institution.

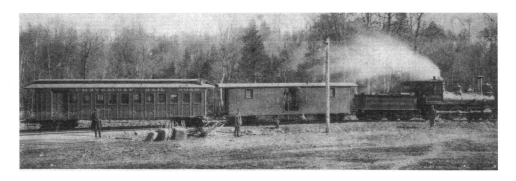

First railway to Saranac Lake
Courtesy of the Trudeau Institute Archives

The Chateaugay Railroad first linked Saranac Lake to the outside world in 1888.

Throughout those years, Dr. Trudeau continued to spend the summers at Paul Smith's where he maintained his medical practice with the guests in and around the neighboring camps. It was his summer practice that helped to meet the growing expenses of his family, as the sanatorium and laboratory contributed no personal financial assistance.

During those summer months, he still journeyed to Saranac Lake by open buggy two days each week for office hours. He would usually arrive by 2 p.m., see patients until 7 p.m., and then begin the arduous fourteen-mile trip back to Paul Smith's. Often upon arrival, he would find the waiting room, lawn, and piazza filled with patients. One day he was presented with a caricature of himself with his patients:

> *I was depicted sitting behind a high picket fence with a double-barreled shot-gun on my lap, waving back an excited crowd who were all shouting impossible questions at me about their health, while underneath was written, "The Penalty of Fame." The thing struck me so funny that I begged it of [my patient], and I still have it as a remembrance of those strenuous office hours.*[57]

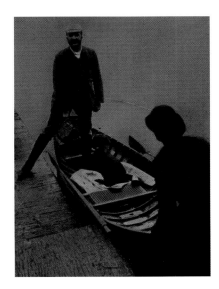

Dr. Trudeau making house calls to the camps in 1894
Courtesy of the Trudeau Institute Archives

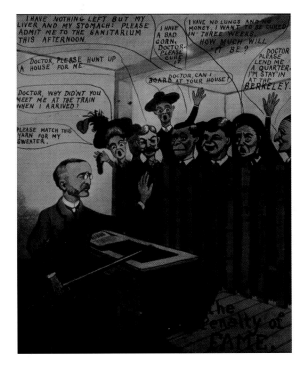

"The Penalty of Fame"
Courtesy of the Trudeau Institute Archives

The years from 1894 to 1906 brought continued growth and development to every department at the sanatorium. Ten new cottages and a water irrigation system had been added. New buildings included a much larger administration building, a nondenominational stone chapel; and Childs Memorial Infirmary, which was "presided over" by Miss Collins. The view from the porch of Childs commanded a magnificent view of the Adirondack Mountains. Patients requiring bed rest were rolled out onto the porch to take their daily treatment of fresh air. According to Trudeau, "It would be hard to find a more attractive place to carry out the doctor's restful sentence."[58]

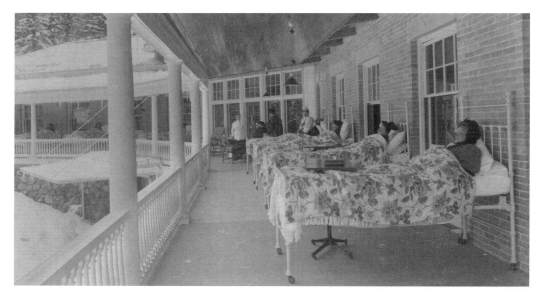
Outdoor cure on the porch of Childs Memorial Infirmary
Courtesy of the Trudeau Institute Archives

The outdoor cure, which had become the mainstay of the treatment regimen at the sanatorium, was defined in the following passage:

> *The invigorating influence of a life spent constantly out of doors for many months can hardly be overrated. To remain, in most cases, the greater part of the time quietly sitting, well wrapped up, out of doors in all weathers, is one of the main duties imposed upon every patient at the sanitarium and, irksome as such a course would at first seem, it is, in a majority of cases, faithfully carried out by them after their timidity and prejudices as to its danger have been gradually overcome by the benefit derived in their own persons.*

> *The outdoor method is applied to all patients, but the details of the treatment, and, above all, the amount of exercise allowed in carrying it out, are regulated by the activity of the patient's disease, his nutritive condition, and more especially his temperature record. Thus, the few*

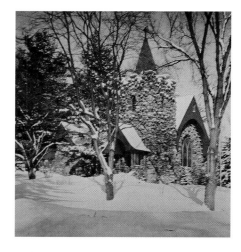
Baker Chapel on grounds of sanatorium
Courtesy of the Trudeau Institute Archives

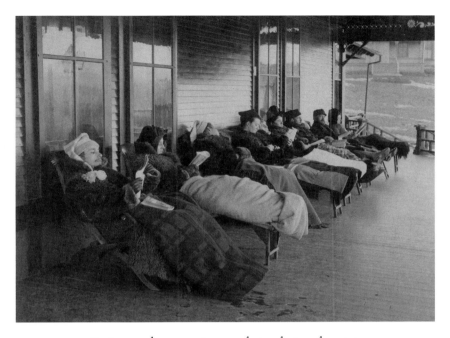

Curing outdoors on steamer chairs during the winter
Courtesy of the Trudeau Institute Archives

infirmary cases who may be suffering from progressive tuberculosis processes or cheesy pneumonias, and running high temperatures, are carried outdoors daily, and kept there in a recumbent position in bed or on a lounge the greater part of the day, while those who have less fever and are improving are allowed to sit up in steamer chairs on the veranda and to walk about the infirmary, but not to go over to their meals in the main building until their temperature record and improved condition warrant it, when they are returned to their cottages. In the class of cases, which is represented by the inmates of the cottages, the temperature rarely goes above a hundred in the afternoon, or they are entirely apyretic. The former are ordered to remain quiet out of doors during the afternoon, when slight fever is apt to occur, and to walk to their meals in the main building, but not to go off the grounds; while the apyretic cases are generally allowed, so long as they live out of doors and obey rules, to go where they please, and while under daily observation, to take as much exercise as their condition seems to render permissible.[59]

The popularity of the outdoor cure was rapidly spreading well beyond the confines of Trudeau's sanatorium on Mt. Pisgah.

The entrepreneurs and healers of Saranac Lake (often in the guise of the same person—a nurse) began to open up houses as private, or non-institutional sanatoria. All but a few of these . . . became virtually synonymous with the term "cure cottages." In a startlingly short time, the movement that had begun with Little Red began to transform the entire village into a cottage sanatorium. It would not be long before the village fathers would begin to publish promotional literature advertising Saranac Lake as the "Pioneer Health Resort" for the treatment of tuberculosis, which in fact it was.[60]

At the turn of the century, about one hundred patients were being cared for at the sanatorium. Many of the patients, desiring to make their cure more permanent, remained on, and sought employment on the grounds. They assisted with the many jobs that were required to run the sanatorium. Similarly, most of the resident physicians were those who needed financial support while they were curing. As they were not interested in the study of tuberculosis for the long term, once their health was sufficiently improved, they moved on. As a result, the administration of the sanatorium was not always efficient and the provision of care was somewhat haphazard.

All this changed in 1901, when Dr. Lawrason Brown became the Resident Physician. His influence upon the institution was immediately evident. The more permissive treatment methodology previously described by Dr. Trudeau soon gave way to Brown's more scrupulous and rigid approach.

> *The essential factors of the sanatorium method of treating tuberculosis I had labored to demonstrate . . . were all generally accepted and permanently established when Dr. Brown became Resident Physician, but the methods were crude, the discipline imperfect, and the records incomplete. The simple and efficient rules of discipline, the thorough instruction of physicians, nurses, and patients, the accurate medical reports and the exhaustive post-discharge records of all patients since the institution started, the Medical Building with its facilities for the careful study of all cases on admission, and another scientific laboratory, all sprang into life as a result of Dr. Brown's insistent efforts for efficiency and continued progress. In addition, he found time to establish and edit for nine years the "Journal of the Outdoor Life," which has rendered such far-reaching service in the crusade against tuberculosis. As I had been only too glad to turn over the Laboratory in Saranac Lake to Dr. Baldwin, it was an immense relief to me to place the medical department of the Sanatorium entirely in Dr. Brown's hands, since soon after his arrival my health and my capacity for work began steadily to fail.[01]*

In 1903 Brown was responsible for originating the first occupational therapy program for tuberculosis patients in the nation. He started the *Journal of the Outdoor Life* in 1904, a magazine specifically for tuberculosis patients that was originally published on the sanatorium's grounds.

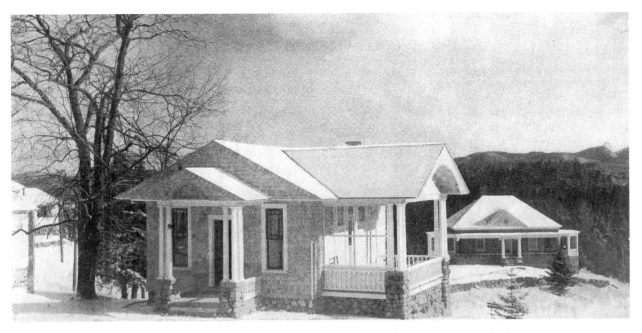

Post office where the "Journal of the Outdoor Life" was also published
Courtesy of the Trudeau Institute Archives

1941 Trudeau, N.Y. postmark
Courtesy of Anne Irene Remis

That same year a post office was established at the sanatorium, and all outgoing mail received the postmark of Trudeau, N.Y. Dr. Brown became the official postmaster and other physicians delivered the mail. The sanatorium was truly becoming a world all its own.

Once again, however, tragedy was about to strike Dr. and Mrs. Trudeau. Ned, the Trudeau's second born child, was a slender but athletic young man who went to Yale University, in New Haven, Connecticut, the fall before Chatte died. Upon graduation from Yale, he attended the College of Physicians and Surgeons. He returned to Saranac Lake after completing his internship at the Presbyterian Hospital in New York City. His father wrote:

He intended to settle here and help me with my work, but I did all I could to dissuade him from this. With his wonderful charm, his very thorough education, and his vigorous health, I saw a much more brilliant future for him elsewhere. I was beginning already to realize the stigma with which the work stamps everything and everybody connected with tuberculosis, and I saw no reason why Ned should voluntarily assume this burden. I was therefore overjoyed when [he was] offered a place in . . . New York City, with every opportunity there for advancement in his profession; and it seemed to me and to all my friends that a very bright future was before him.[62]

Perhaps his son could now realize "the rose-colored dreams" of achievement and professional success in New York that were denied Dr. Trudeau so many years before. Ned soon married, and at the reception Dr. Trudeau could not help thinking:

What a brilliant future was before him, for in addition to his personal advantages, he had already many warm friends in New York among the very best people there, and his connection with Dr. James gave him a wonderful opportunity in his professional life. I rejoiced then I had not let him assume a more obscure career with his father in the remote little Adirondack village, with its ever-present burden of chronic illness.[63]

How quickly everything changed. In the spring of 1904, the Trudeaus received a telegram from Dr. Walter B. James telling them that Ned had suddenly contracted acute lobar pneumonia and to come immediately. After five days Ned was through the crisis. But just as the Trudeaus were able to breathe a huge sigh of relief over his apparent recovery, Ned died suddenly of a pulmonary embolism.

I cannot write about his death. My wife and I passed through days of dazed suffering, which even now it is hard to dwell upon and from which we have never recovered, for life has never been the same to us since.

Through all these terrible, dark days, however, the tender sympathy and love of our friends and his friends shone, and shines even now, like a soft light in the midst of impenetrable gloom. Everyone who knew Ned and knew us tried to show their love for him, and that touched us and helped us bear our own suffering. I cannot write it all, but the full record is written so deep in our hearts that nothing can ever dim it.

The next afternoon at the Grand Central Station we found two cars Mr. [Edward H.] Harriman had arranged for, attached to the Adirondack train. In one Ned's body lay, buried under a roomful of flowers and surrounded by his Yale chums, who sat up all night by him as the car sped through the darkness toward the mountains and the little churchyard under the tall pines at Paul Smith's. The other car was prepared for us and many friends.

The next morning broke clear and beautiful, and as we approached the Church it was evident the whole country had come to show their love for the young man who had lived his boyhood and most of his life among them. . . . Paul Smith and his sons and other faithful friends had covered all the ground from the Church to the grave with flowers and green boughs. . . . Had Ned been their own son and brother they could not have done more.

But I was to have further proof of the love and esteem in which he was held. A few days later I started out to collect and settle all the bills for the funeral. Everywhere the answer was the same. There was no bill. What they had done, they had done for him.[04]

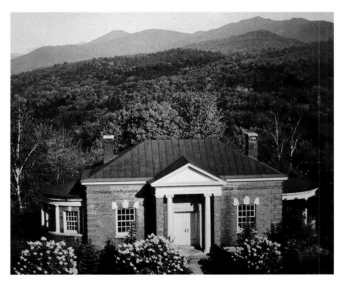

Mellon Library
Courtesy of the Trudeau Institute Archives

The humility, that was so much a part of Dr. Trudeau, blinded him to the true message behind such magnanimous gestures. What they had done was only in part done for Ned. There could be little doubt that this overwhelming gift of love was even more a tribute to Dr. and Mrs. Trudeau who had given so selflessly, continuously, and unconditionally in the twenty-eight years they had lived in this small community. Finally, during their darkest hours, the little village could give back to the two individuals responsible for its very creation.

And despite Dr. Trudeau's worsening health from 1904 to 1915, the sanatorium continued to grow and flourish. By 1914 the endowment had grown to $600,000 and the Free Bed Fund, first established in 1888, continued to grow and provide free care to many patients unable to contribute toward their stay. More cottages were built, as was a library, a reception and medical building, and a workshop building for occupational therapy.

Over the years, Trudeau credited the success of the sanatorium to many people. At the close of his autobiography, he offered sincere thanks to the trustees, the physicians, the superintendents and their helpers, the nurses, and even the employees who often worked without pay; all of whom contributed to the material and financial success of the institution. In 1884 his had become the first sanatorium of its kind for the treatment of tuberculosis in the United States. By 1909, three hundred fifty-two private and state institutions for the treatment of tuberculosis had followed Trudeau's model.

On February 15, 1910, Dr. Trudeau celebrated the sanatorium's twenty-fifth anniversary. He was presented with a leather-bound book, made in the sanatorium workshop, that contained congratulatory cards from 1,000 former patients whose lives his treatments had prolonged. In his address on that eventful day, Trudeau, filled with emotion, spoke the following words:

> How can I find words to express suitably my feelings on such an occasion as this? Twenty-five years ago I dreamed a dream, and, lo, it has come true, and we are here today to commemorate the realization of this dream.

> When I came to the Adirondacks thirty-five years ago the outlook for my accomplishing anything in life seemed to be hopeless indeed. I was an exile in a country, which was both remote and inaccessible. I had only an indifferent medical education . . . I had only ordinary intellectual attainments. Now you may ask how it was, in spite of these difficulties, I accomplished what has been done here.

> The first asset I had, which carried me through better than anything else, was a good wife— the best wife that any man ever had; and through the long years of discouragement and struggle she has always furnished both inspiration and encouragement. And then I had an unlimited fund of enthusiasm and perseverance, and I had faith; that kind of faith that sees the goal and is blind to the obstacles; faith in myself; faith in my power to do something, no matter how little, for a good cause; faith in my friends—and that faith has been reflected on me so that they have poured their money into my lap all these years for my work; faith in the future, here and hereafter.

Now that I have come to the end of the road, what more could I ask than to be permitted to stand with you here today and see the realization of my dream; . . to stand here and see those who have been connected with this work for so many years—doctors, nurses, and those in the administration department. . . . And what is better than to see all about me those whose lives have been saved and prolonged, and to know that this saving and prolonging of life, because of what we have striven to do here all these years, has reached across the continent and brought hope and life to those who hitherto were hopeless.[05]

In his last years, it was increasingly difficult for Dr. Trudeau to get around. His faithful guide, Fitz, did not want to see the day come when his hunting companion could no longer enjoy his favorite pastime in the woods. Therefore, Fitz, in all his ingenuity, fashioned various conveyances that could be used to carry the doctor into the woods for his hunts.

One of Trudeau's last proud accomplishments was the establishment of a training school for nurses. The school was started in 1912, for the purpose of:

Dr. and Mrs. Trudeau
Courtesy of the Trudeau Institute Archives

educating as special tuberculosis nurses some of the young women patients in whom the Sanitarium treatment had arrested the disease, and thus fit them for an independent career of usefulness which does not especially endanger their health. It is a far cry from the old women and guides I used to hire to do the nursing of the bedridden in the first years of the Sanitarium, to a graduating class of thoroughly trained nurses such as I had before me when I handed the diplomas on both these occasions to the graduates. . . . These nurses readily find employment in Saranac Lake, or take up institutional work elsewhere.[66]

And so it finally came to pass, that at 11:40 a.m. on a dreary day in November of 1915, the man, who for forty-three years had refused to die, quietly surrendered to the disease he had spent so long trying to conquer. Edward Livingston Trudeau was finally laid to rest beside baby Henry, Chatte, and Ned beneath the tall pines near the eaves of the little church that he had helped to build nearly forty years before.

The Adirondack Cottage Sanitarium was renamed the Trudeau Sanatorium in 1917. The Trudeau influence continued to flourish. That same year a post-graduate school for physicians to receive six-week training in tuberculosis was begun. Many physicians from around the world were drawn to the area in order to take advantage of the educational opportunities that were available at the sanatorium.

More than seven years after the death of her husband, Mrs. Trudeau, the woman who was always at her husband's side, died at her home in Saranac Lake on February 23, 1923. Her friend, Dr. Allen Kraus, described Mrs. Trudeau as:

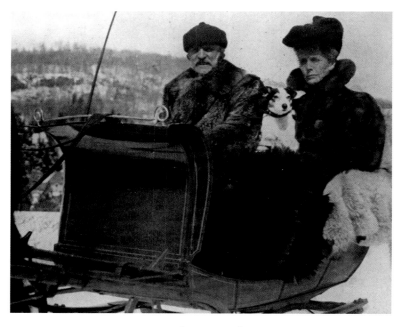

Dr. and Mrs. Trudeau
Courtesy of the Trudeau Institute Archives

> *a polite, refined, and elegant woman who gave up everything that was dear to her in life— everything but her husband—[and] entered upon the great experiment with him. Gracious to a degree, she was gifted with a strength of character, a spiritual strength, that was her outstanding trait. Quiet, restrained and deep, she was a perfect counterpart to her scintillating, talkative and animated husband. The doctor's emotions lay near the surface and would now and then blaze up, and at critical times threaten to unnerve. But at these times "Lottie" was always the rock, fixed and stable, and a secure refuge. Her deep and tranquil sympathy steadied him during his many periods of illness and buoyed him wonderfully when he began to see darkly.*[67]

After the service, which was held at St. Luke's Church in Saranac Lake, the funeral procession drove through Trudeau Sanatorium for what was said to be the most impressive part of the service.

The bell in the little chapel that Dr. Trudeau had founded, and in which Mrs. Trudeau had taken such an active interest, tolled. The patients and nurses gathered on the porch of the main building as the procession passed. The patients unable to walk stood in front of their own cottages. It was the final tribute to the helpmate of the illustrious man who had made the sanatorium, the first of its kind in America, possible.[68]

Forty-eight years earlier, when Mrs. Trudeau first came into the woods, the snow was up to the shoulders of their horses and a small cave had to be dug into the snow for shelter. When Chatte was buried, recall that the snow was four feet deep and it took six men to steady her little coffin as the horses again struggled through the drifts. And now, Mrs. Trudeau's final journey also ended as it began. Starting out by train, the sleighs finished the balance of the journey from Saranac Lake to St. John's in the Wilderness in St. Regis. The snows, one last time, rose to four feet almost as though to pay final tribute to the passing of this proud woman whose death signaled the end of an era. Although the snow about the little church was drifted to four feet, the entire yard was shoveled by hand and the five graves of the Trudeau family were uncovered, clear to the ground.

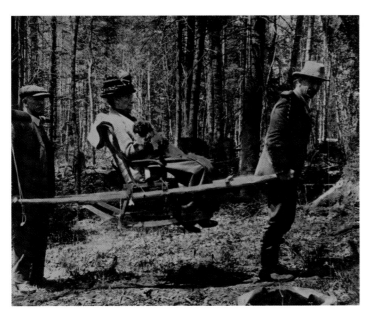

Mrs. Trudeau in one of the hunting chairs made by Fitz, their guide and companion
Courtesy of the Trudeau Institute Archives

The church was thrown open as in mid-summer. A fire was roaring in the furnace, but the windows and doors were wide open. The altar was prepared just as Mrs. Trudeau had so often prepared it with her own hands for the services.[69]

Family, friends, employees, and several of the nurses, guides and their families gathered at the church to bid their final good-by. Mrs. Trudeau joined her husband and three children beneath the tall pines near the eaves of the little church that her husband had built nearly fifty years before.

Dr. Francis B. Trudeau, the last-born child of Dr. and Mrs. Trudeau, continued his father's work at the sanatorium until its closing in 1954. Like his father, Dr. Francis, who was described by one of his closest associates "as one of the kindest men I have ever known," also had a deep love and reverence for the outdoors:

> He not only loved the majesty of the hills and the serenity of the lakes and streams. He loved to do the things that the hills, lakes and streams made possible. To walk and to climb. To fish and to hunt.

> He cherished the flowers and the trees, knew them, talked about them, collected them. He knew the birds and the animals.

> But he knew also the sense of divinity which is in nature, and this perception of nature's great mystery was, we would venture to guess, the most penetrating influence in his life.[70]

And on a magnificent Adirondack summer day in July of 1956, when the air was warm and fresh and tangy, Dr. Francis, who was enjoying an early afternoon boat ride on St. Regis Lake, turned to his wife who was behind him in a smaller boat, slumped forward and died. Amid unsurpassed beauty and tranquility, Nature gave to one of its own the gift of a painless passing.

His son, Dr. Francis B. Trudeau, Jr., had the same vision and pioneering spirit as did his grandfather. His philosophy was similar to that of his grandfather, who had a very altruistic approach to the practice of medicine. Like his father and his grandfather, he was said to be a man of overwhelming kindness and gentleness. Wanting to carry on in the traditions of his ancestors, Dr. Francis, Jr., founded the Trudeau Institute, a world-class center for basic research in immunology and infectious disease, on Lower Saranac Lake. Dr. Francis Trudeau, Jr., said he wanted to create an institute:

> that provided an optimal contemplative environment for the pursuit of research, that stood alone, unencumbered by administrative duties of the politics of a university, with the freedom to do research whenever you wish.[71]

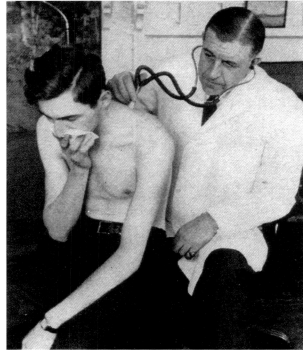

Dr. Francis B. Trudeau in 1937
Alfred Eisenstadt/TimePix

The Scientist ranked the Trudeau Institute seventh on a list of twenty high-impact independent biological and biomedical research institutions in the United States. Dr. Francis Trudeau, Jr., who was the third and last physician in the family since his grandfather moved to the area, died on April 25, 1995, leaving behind his second wife, Ursula Wyatt Trudeau. He also left a son, Garry, the creator of the *Doonesbury* comic strip; two daughters, Jeanne Fenn, a photographer; and Michelle Trudeau, a correspondent for National Public Radio; and their mother, Jean Amory of Vero Beach, Florida.[72]

Trudeau Institute has continued to attract highly trained scientists from around the world. Although the research tools they use have changed, their spirit of adventure and goal of service have not. E. L. Trudeau would surely recognize these as the legacy he left science and the world.[73]

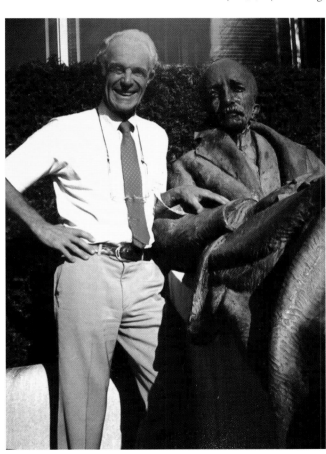

Dr. Francis B. Trudeau, Jr., standing next to the statue of his grandfather on the grounds of the Trudeau Institute. It overlooks the mountains rising above Lower Saranac Lake.
Courtesy of Lilo Levine

Our Physician
*Of infinite compassion, vision keen,
Great mind and greater heart—of purpose high
That lifts his work to heights of majesty
Above all motives commonplace or mean;
His life is pledged to combat. As of old
Fought Arthur and his knights against the sway
Of murderous hordes, he strives to keep at bay
A foe more deadly, pitiless and bold,
That spoils our land, and no condition spares,
The changing seasons mark his changeless aim,
Highest and lowest alike acclaim
Their champion, as steadfastly he fares,
Unresting, self-regardless, on his quest,
By all who know him, loved, revered and blessed.
~Charlotte Stuart Best, 1925*

The Hills of Trudeau

There's a mist upon the mountains, there's rain among the hills,
The valleys of the meadow lands are gray;
The snows of half the winter are singing in the rills,
And every clod is quivering for May.
There are buds that swell to bursting and birds in every glen,
There's a miracle abroad upon the land.
There's a vast, entrancing beauty to feast the eyes of men—
When comes it, and at whose august command?
There's a spirit in the mountains, a courage in the air,
There's a greatness, and a majesty that thrills;
There is hope and healing wisdom, and joy for those who dare—
O Trudeau. There is God among thy hills!

~Mrs. L. Rice, 1907

University of Hope:
Portrait of a Patient

*I*f Saranac Lake could be called the "University of Tuberculosis,"[1] then the microcosm among the sick that was so rapidly developing on the side of Mt. Pisgah could surely be called the "University of Hope." What started out as one building on sixteen acres of land had, by 1951, mushroomed into fifty-eight buildings that spread across eighty-five acres. Thirty years after its inception, as Trudeau described the changes that had taken place, it could easily have been mistaken for a university.

The mountains now look down on a different scene. The old boulders and the rough pasture have disappeared, and macadamized roads, sloping grass lawns, flower

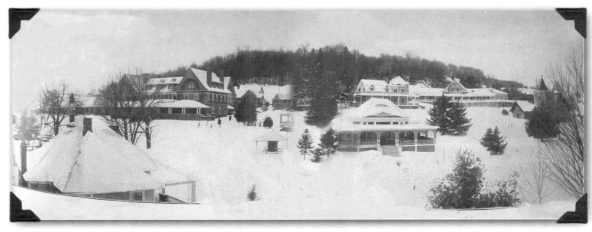

Trudeau Sanatorium in 1930
Courtesy of the Trudeau Institute Archives

beds and ornamental shrubs have taken their place. The Sanitarium has grown to be a picturesque little village. It comprises thirty-six buildings scattered over the entire hillside between the north and south gates, a distance of about three quarters of a mile. The patients' cottages are grouped about the large Administration Building and other cottages for the heads of departments are clustered together at the south entrance, near which are the stables, barns, and the big fire-proof laundry. In addition to the patients' cottages, there are many other buildings which represent various activities: a nurses' home for the Training School, an infirmary for bed-ridden patients, a post office, a colonial brick and marble library building, a reception and medical building with offices, laboratory and x-ray department, a recreating pavilion for amusements and entertainments, a workshop building where the patients are taught fancy leather-work, book-binding, brass work and frame-making as a recreation and as graded exercise, and a beautiful stone chapel.[2]

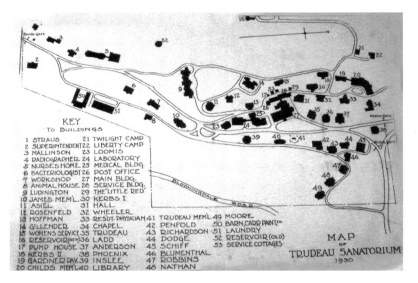

1930 Map of Trudeau Sanatorium
Courtesy of the Trudeau Institute Archives

Prior to Trudeau, who turned tuberculosis from a "malady to a career;"[3] the disease was thought to guarantee its victim a death sentence. Charles Dickens, in *Nicholas Nickleby*, offered a haunting description of the disease:

There is a dread disease which so prepared its victim, as it were, for death; which so refines it of grosser aspects, and throws around it unearthly indications of the coming change—a dread disease in which the struggle between soul and body is so gradual, quiet and solemn, and the result so sure, that day by day and grain by grain the mortal part wastes and withers away, so that the spirit grows light and sanguine with its lightening load, and, feeling mortality at hand, deems it but a new term of mortal life; a disease in which death and life are so strangely blended that death takes the hue of life and life the gaunt and grisly form of death; a disease which medicine never cured, wealth never warded off or poverty could boast exemption from; which sometimes moves in giant strides and sometimes at a tardy sluggish pace, but, slow or quick, is ever sure and certain.[4]

But Trudeau's University of Hope offered to the patients fortunate enough to gain entry more than a commutation from that death sentence. Newly diagnosed patients arriving at the gates of Trudeau Sanatorium were heavily burdened with the knowledge that they had contracted the disease that almost certainly signaled impending death. Yet again and again, past patients recall how their feelings of doom and despair were instantly replaced by feelings of hope and optimism as soon as they walked through those gates. The months and years spent at the sanatorium were described as life transforming. Today, numerous sanatorium "graduates" emphatically state that TB was the best thing that ever happened to them. What was it about this remarkable institution that caused its "alumni" to move back in for summer retreats once they had been cured and discharged? What was it about the TB experience that made people want to meet years later on the streets of Saranac Lake to celebrate TB reunions? And why is it, that nearly fifty years after its closing, many of those who cured at this sanatorium still look lovingly at their scrapbooks filled with mementoes from their years of healing? To answer these questions, let us take a glimpse at what life was like on the inside of this "university."

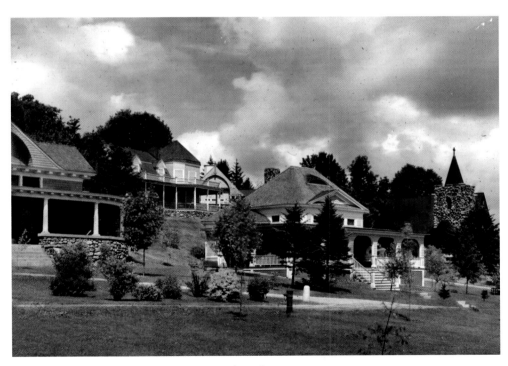

Expansion of Trudeau Sanatorium
Courtesy of the Trudeau Institute Archives

Where once the hospital had been a place of horror, a repository for the hopeless . . . the sanatorium transformed it into an extension of everyday life, a place where living, albeit tubercular living, went on much as it did everywhere. If to the cynical observer its completeness in isolation and its self-sufficiency might suggest a leper colony, for the patient it proved that he was not cut off from the world, only leading a parallel life in special circumstances.[5]

Admission Requirements

The two prime entry requirements were curability of disease and financial resources that could not otherwise meet the cost of care elsewhere. In the *Second Annual Report of The Adirondack Cottage Sanitarium*, the following rules applied to admission of patients:

Class of Patients

Only those who are in the first stages of consumption or convalescing from other pulmonary diseases—who can go about freely to enjoy the pure air—and whose circumstances are such as to admit of their paying only the low price demanded here for board are admitted to the cottages.

Admission

All applicants for admission to cottages, from a distance, must be examined by Dr. A. L. Loomis, personally, and have a written certificate of suitability as a patient from him addressed to Dr. Trudeau, or they will not be admitted. Those nearer the cottages may apply directly to Dr. Trudeau for admission.

All applicants to either Drs. Loomis or Trudeau must have a letter from their home physician certifying to the genuineness of their application, when they will be examined free of charge, otherwise the regular fee for examination will be charged.

Cost to Patients

Drs. Loomis, Trudeau, and Wicker, of Saranac Lake, N.Y. give their services free of cost to all patients.

Five dollars per week is charged for board and lodging.

Fifty cents per dozen pieces for washing.

There are no extra charges whatever.

Friends coming with or visiting patients, can not remain longer than one week, and will be charged one dollar per day.

All medicines can be procured at village drug stores at a discount. A number of medicines are kept at Cottages and furnished at cost to patients.[6]

Trudeau tried to limit his admissions to incipient cases as they had the greatest chance of a cure. In 1898 he published treatment results of 203 patients in his annual report. After a stay of nine months, seventy-three percent of his incipient cases were apparently cured with no reported deaths. Only eighteen percent of his advanced cases were apparently cured with only one reported death. Of those that were considered to be far advanced cases, zero percent were apparently cured during the same length of stay, and eleven percent died.[7] Upon discharge, patients were termed "apparently cured" once they had maintained a normal life-style for two years without relapse.

In a later report, Trudeau discussed the results of Dr. Lawrason Brown's study of 1,500 cases:

> 434 could not be traced, leaving 1066 which have been traced. Of these 46.7 percent are living. Of these 31 percent are known to be well at present, in 6.5 percent the disease is still arrested, 4 percent have relapsed, 5.2 percent are chronic invalids, and 53.3 percent are dead. As to the influence of the stage of the disease on the permanency of the results obtained, he found 66 percent of the 258 incipient cases discharged are well at present. Of the 563 advanced cases 28.6 percent are well, and of the far advanced cases 2.5 percent only, remain well.

> These figures, discouraging as they may seem to those of you who are not familiar with this fatal malady, emphasize the importance of making an early diagnosis, and teach us exactly to what extent we may count on saving and prolonging life by this method of treatment.[8]

These statistics confirmed to Trudeau the importance of early discovery and provided justification for admitting primarily patients who were in the incipient stages of the disease and were, therefore, more amenable to a cure. In the hopes of increasing secondary levels of prevention, Trudeau widely disseminated the following clues, which suggested incipient stage disease, to his referring physicians:

> In insidious cases lassitude, some loss of appetite, a little quickening of the pulse-rate, a temperature reaching occasionally 99.5 to 100 degrees at irregular intervals, with or without slight loss of weight, are a group of symptoms which usually attracts little attention, but which should be regarded with suspicion. And if, in addition to these, morning pallor, disappearing toward evening, some cough, prolonged expiration, or even impairment of vesicular murmur are noted, the patient should be closely

watched, every effort made to obtain more positive evidence; and if it's not obtainable otherwise, the aid of laboratory methods in helping to clear up the diagnosis should not be neglected.[9]

Gradually the word spread that Trudeau's sanatorium treatment could offer hope, often in the name of cure, to those lucky enough to be eligible for admission. Furthermore, soon after admission to the sanatorium, patients discovered that their cure included a variety of educational opportunities; many of which were far from traditional course offerings.

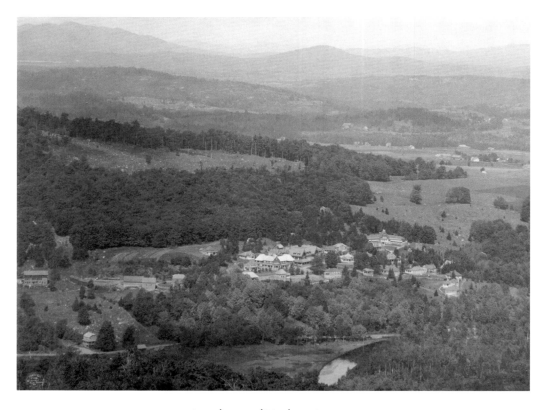

Aerial view of Trudeau Sanatorium
Courtesy of the Trudeau Institute Archives

The sanatorium offered more than hope for recovery; it was also becoming the pioneer educational institution in the tuberculosis movement. Many of the educational programs that were so much a part of the sanatorium somehow instilled in each patient a strong desire to tap the full potential of their creativity and talent that the disease of tuberculosis seemed to unleash.

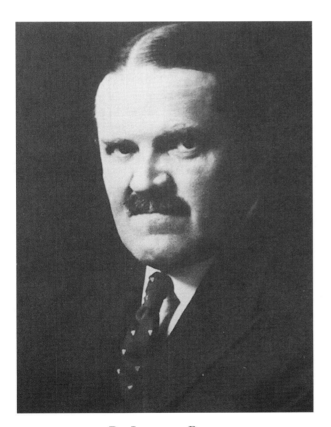

Dr. Lawrason Brown
Courtesy of the Trudeau Institute Archives

Numerous patients have spoken of the heightened creativity that seemed almost symptomatic of the disease. One nurse who cured and nursed at the sanatorium, when asked what she thought contributed to the heightened creativity that accompanied the disease, responded, "I think it had a lot to do with serenity, and that their minds had to become active because their bodies were so repressed. They had to for survival. They couldn't use their bodies so all their energy went to their mental processes."[10]

Occupational Therapy

Dr. Lawrason Brown was the educational architect behind much of the innovative programming that was developing at the sanatorium. His genius was given encouragement and free rein by Dr. Trudeau, always the altruist, whose goal was not the need to receive personal credit for innovation, but rather to encourage any ideas that had the potential for achieving positive patient outcomes.

Dr. Allen Krause, a long time friend and colleague of Dr. Trudeau, had the following to say in his reminiscences of the sanatorium and Dr. Brown:

The Trudeau Sanatorium is the living symbol of Trudeau, and is his monument. Beautiful in form, and well balanced and complete in plan and equipment, it still follows the best canons of practice and of study and through it all runs a broad and deep current of humanity. It also envisages all that was great and good in the doctor. Happily, before he closed his eyes, it was granted him to gaze upon a scene and view a work that must have far outshone the most golden dreams of the lone fox-hunter on Pisgah's runway. And it must not be forgotten that he once put a young Baltimore doctor there, and that this Lawrason Brown is the man who, through a long tenure of residence, may be called the master-builder of Trudeau's Sanatorium, the fashioner of its larger plan.[11]

Dr. Brown, a scholarly man with a passion for organization, was remembered as:

an owlish, taciturn and rather untidy figure; plagued by foot trouble, he used to shuffle in bedroom slippers through the streets and into the sickrooms of his patients, on whom, however unprepossessing his appearance, he had an uplifting effect.[12]

Brown believed that "the success of a physician in treating pulmonary tuberculosis depends largely on his ability to deal skillfully and individually with the physical, psychological, and sociological problems that arise with each patient. His former habits, pursuits, and idiosyncrasies must be carefully noted."[13] He certainly paid heed to his owns words for the success of Brown's "experiment" in 1903 was undisputed and of far reaching historical significance.

In 1903 Dr. Trudeau put before his Board of Trustees Dr. Brown's idea of some sort of occupation for the patients.

For a long time there has been a great need of some co-operative system that would furnish the patients whose disease has been arrested suitable employment and surroundings where they might do enough work to support themselves for sometime after their discharge from the Sanitarium and until their restoration to health may be more permanently established. An effort to solve this difficult problem, and to obtain suitable employment for as many as possible, will be attempted this year as an experiment.[14]

Dr. Brown, bothered by ongoing patient complaints of "ennui," devised an intriguing solution in the name of Herbert Scholfield and Occupational Therapy.

Some twenty years previously, [in 1884], [Herbert Scholfield] had been sent as a boy to the Adirondacks, where he had taught school and better still had schooled himself in resignation to the inevitable, for he realized that he would never be well, and had devoted himself to high ideals. He was skilled in many handicrafts, and at this time he had built a kiln and was firing his own handmade pottery. And so to this man of many resources, ennui was unknown, and his experience had led him to treat the many patients protesting against their limitations, with the indulgence that an affectionate mother gives her petulant children. We talked over the problem that I had to face in the Sanatorium and the possibility of giving the patients something to occupy their leisure time. I then placed the plan before Dr. Trudeau with the result that we remodeled the Lea Cottage into an open-air workshop for tuberculosis patients, the first in America. Here with the assistance of Mr. Perkins, who designed a work table heated by an oil lamp, which enabled patients to work out of doors without gloves in all save the bitterest weather, Mr. Scholfield began his real life work. He taught bookbinding, leatherwork, woodcarving, illuminating, and from time to time added new crafts. From this time I had no more complaints of ennui from the patients.

Mr. Scholfield had the privilege of taking private pupils from the village of Saranac Lake and charging them, for his salary was in keeping with those paid the other workers. Even so, time and again, he spent part of his meager income on some new device, for the blood of his ancestors who introduced knitting into New England ran strong in his veins. One day an attractive woman, a lover and collector of books, a patient of Dr. Trudeau's, sought private instruction, learned how to bind books, and having recovered her health and about to leave, asked Mr. Scholfield for his bill. His greatest pleasure was to teach those who loved the things he loved. His open-air workshop was at that time his

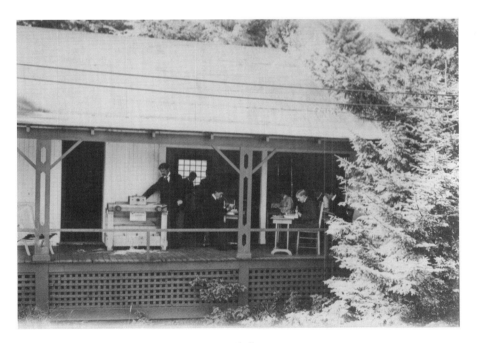

Open-Air Workshop in 1904
Courtesy of the Trudeau Institute Archives

whole life, and he told her he wanted nothing for himself but that she could give something for the shop. Pausing for a moment, she replied, "I will give you a new workshop." Idealism, self-denial, altruism, had won out. Mrs. Goodwin, now Mrs. Frances Hare, built the splendid workshop we now have at Trudeau, and gave to Mr. Scholfield the greatest happiness of his life, and to many patients, tired and weary of reading and sitting, a safe outlet for energy, an introduction to many beautiful things of life which before they looked upon but saw not.[15]

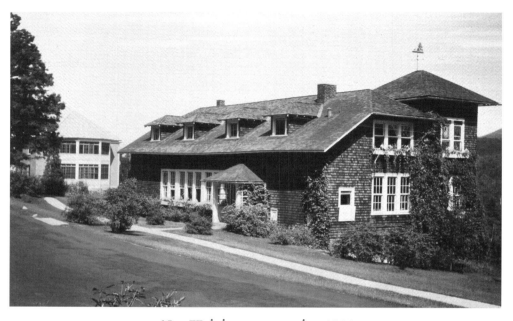

New Workshop constructed in 1909
Courtesy of the Trudeau Institute Archives

The true origin of occupational therapy remains open for some dispute. Numerous sources credit Dr. Brown for its birth at the Adirondack Cottage Sanitarium in 1904. A more accurate statement would be to credit Dr. Brown, certainly as the first who created the concept of outdoor occupational therapy, and likely the first to utilize occupational therapy with tuberculosis patients, and perhaps the first to use occupational therapy with patients who were mentally well. The actual origin of using this type of therapy on a patient population came well before Dr. Brown's time.

One hundred years before the birth of Christ, there was evidence of the use of therapeutic baths, massage, exercise, and music in the treatment of patients with mental illness. At the turn of the twentieth century, the idea of work as a therapeutic component in the treatment of people with mental disorders was revived. The Hull House in Chicago, which was founded by Jane Addams and Ellen Gates Starr in 1889, provided community services and recreation to the poor. The Chicago Arts and Crafts Society was organized at Hull House in 1897.

[There, many Chicagoans] participated in this larger American and British movement by studying a variety of arts and crafts processes and thus resisting what they perceived to be the tyranny of the machine. . . . Craftwork . . . provided opportunities for them as non-working-class people to capture what they perceived to be a productive and meaningful life experience. By actually using their hands, creating specimens of pottery, wood, glass, metal, or cloth, the members hoped to gain insight into the problem with which they struggled incessantly—alienation in modern life.[16]

In 1892, Dr. Adolph Meyer, a psychiatrist, reported that using time in gratifying and useful ways appeared to be helpful when dealing with the neuropsychiatric patient. Further, in 1895, William Rush Dunton, Jr., a psychiatrist in Baltimore, used metalworking with his psychiatric patients; and Mary Potter Brooks Meyer introduced systematic activity into the wards of a state institution in Worchester, Massachusetts.[17]

The actual meaning of the word "occupational" when used in conjunction with the word therapy is subject to various interpretations. During the early part of 1910, many interpreted the word to mean "vocational" dealing specifically with learning a new occupation. Later, with the first generation of occupational therapists, it took on a more expanded interpretation.

They took a holistic approach to health care, believing that to achieve good health, a patient had to engage body, mind, and spirit in the process of healing. Healing . . . came about when patients were "occupied" with work, in particular, with craft activity. By interacting with individual patients and by observing with their own eyes, the early occupational therapists learned that occupational therapy restored physical function, improved mental attitude, and in general, lessened suffering, thus quickening convalescence.[18]

Susan E. Tracy, who organized occupational therapy classes in her training school for nurses at the Adams Nervine Asylum in 1906, was considered to be the first occupational therapist. However, as the work of Dr. Brown, with his occupational therapy experiment with tuberculosis patients in 1903 to 1904, predates the work of Susan Tracy and others, there is some merit to sources that credit Brown with the birth of modern occupational therapy.

Perhaps the question of who was first is of small importance. What is significant, however, is that the Adirondack Cottage Sanitarium, hidden away in a remote and tiny village in the Adirondacks, was on the cutting edge of a new treatment modality. There is no question that Brown's use of Occupational Therapy was both vocational and occupational and, most certainly, it was both a form of therapy and education.

Although most of the sanitaria in existence at the turn of the century offered some form of amusement to occupy the patient's time, the most unique was the extensive system of combined therapy and instruction that was developing at the Adirondack Cottage Sanitarium.

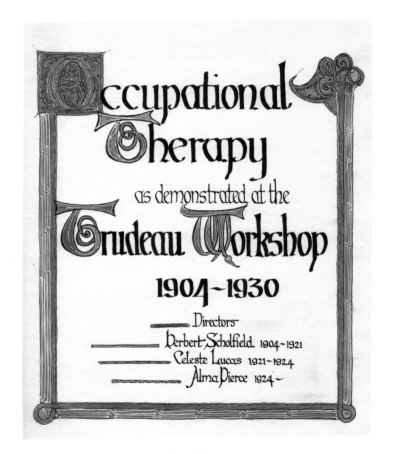

> *Regular class work in stenography and telegraphy is maintained throughout the year. Classes in botany and in the study of bird life are conducted during the warmer months. . . . There is no charge for instruction.*
>
> *The distinctive feature of the educational work at this sanatorium is the Phoenix Workshop. . . . The outer room where most of the operations in picture-framing and bookbinding are done is entirely open on one side so that one works practically out-of-doors. During the colder months of the year the work-table in this room is warmed by hot-water pipes. For the more delicate work, like lettering and illuminating, individual desks are provided on the partially glazed veranda. . . . Work can be carried on even during the winter months, provided the worker is clothed as warmly as for "taking the cure," and the temperature is not so low (about 10 degrees Fahrenheit) as to freeze the ink on the pen and the water-color in the brush before it can be put to paper. The warmed desk is quite sufficient to keep one's fingers from getting numb and one's materials from freezing. . . . Some of the work done by Mr. Scholfield and his pupils . . . compare favorably with such work done anywhere in America.*[19]

Example of illumination
Courtesy of Trudeau Institute Archives

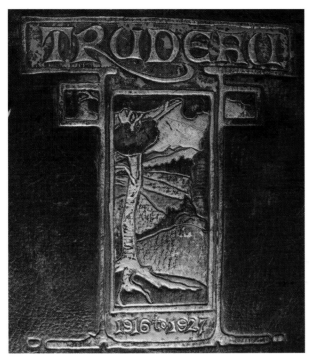

Tooled leather scrapbook cover made in
Trudeau Workshop

The photographs on the following
pages were located in a scrapbook
entitled: "Patient Workshops,
1904-1930,"
in the archive collection at the
Trudeau Institute.

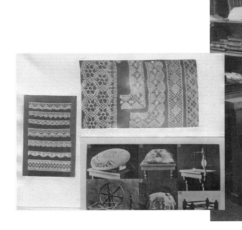

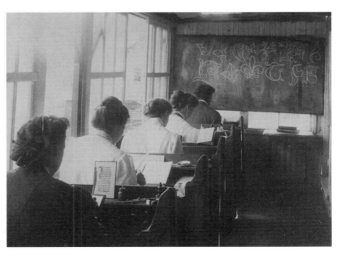

Mr. Scholfield making lace

Learning illumination in the Open-Air
Workshop. Note the open windows on
the left.

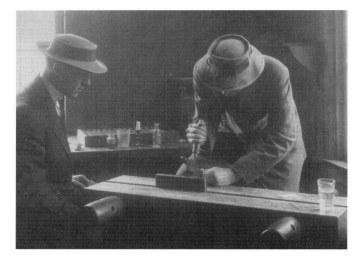

Putting gold title on a book

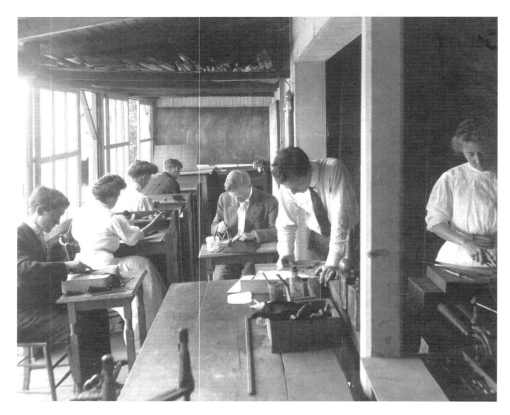

Learning bookbinding in Open-Air Workshop in 1886

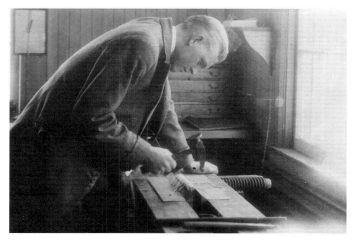

Backing a book

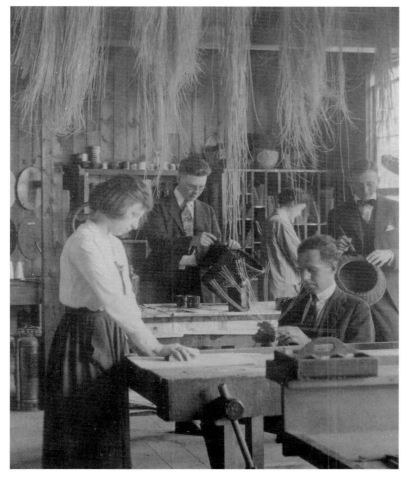

Basketry

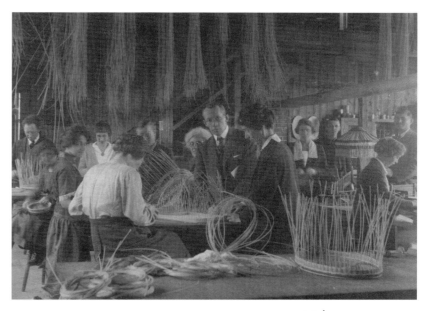

Making a tea tray

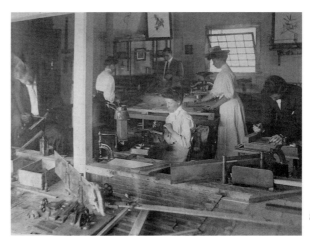

Occupational therapy activities in 1908

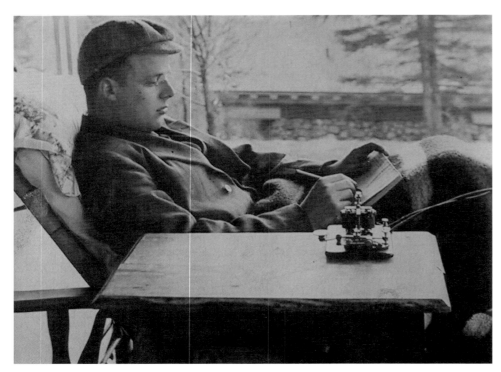

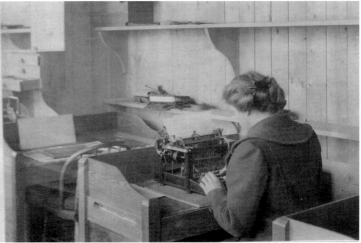

Learning to type in 1918

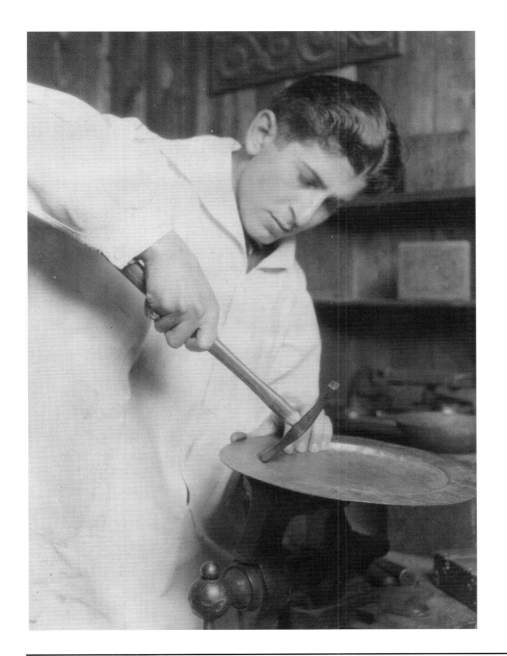

Mr. Ensler making a copper plate

Batiks made in 1929

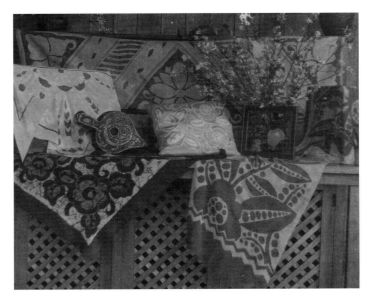

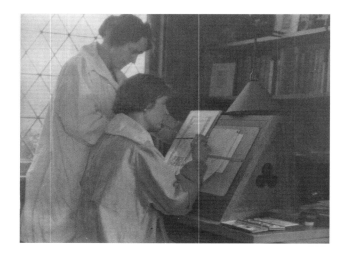

Miss Pierce, a former patient, teaching illuminating

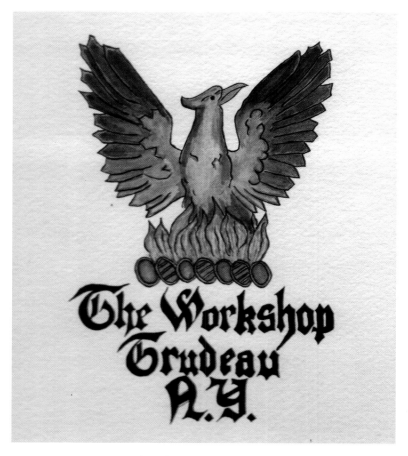

The Phoenix Workshop logo

In 1935 the Saranac Lake Study and Craft Guild was established in the village by some of the doctors and ex-patients as a result of the huge popularity of the occupational therapy program at the sanatorium. The Guild was supported by the state, private contributions, and small fees from the pupils who could afford to pay. It developed into a thriving rehabilitation center for those confined to bed as well as for those who were slowly regaining their health. Training courses were offered in more than sixty subjects. The Guild enabled many high school students, who were confined to bed rest, to continue their schoolwork so that they could qualify for college despite their illness. One of the Guild specialties was the training of ex-tuberculosis patients to become x-ray operators for the public-health mobile detection unit that traveled throughout the country in search of tuberculosis. It was the individuals who first had received training in Saranac Lake that were later responsible for staffing nearly every mobile unit in the country.

Dr. Brown established a magazine for TB patients in 1904, called the *Outdoor Life*, later called *Journal of the Outdoor Life*, which he edited for nine years. It was printed on the grounds of the sanatorium until it was later taken over by the National Tuberculosis Association and moved to its new headquarters in New York City. In the first issue of February 1904, Dr. Trudeau included the following words in the Foreword:

> As "Outdoor Life" starts out on its career it has my heartiest approval and best wishes. I hope that it may prove a link that will bind together friendship begun while living the out-of-doors life, that it will instruct all the disciples of this life as to the best methods of getting the best results mentally and physically from an out-of-door life and that it will bring something of the freshness, hope and vigor of this out-of-door life to many poor indoor mortals who know nothing of its benefits and pleasures.[20]

Dr. Brown, as the editor, contributed the following:

> It is usual when a new periodical makes its first appearance to devote some of its space to an explanation of what it is. Such an explanation it is hoped is unnecessary in this case, but a word or two in regards the aims of the "Outdoor Life" may be of interest. As the name signifies this paper will be published in the interests of those who either for pleasure or for health are leading more or less of an outdoor life. Its constant aim will be to suggest how to get the most pleasure or the most health, or better, how to combine both in and outdoor life. No detail that will add some comfort will be considered too small to bring to the attention of our readers. Suggestions along this line will always be given the space that is due them. It is hoped that from time to time we shall be able to publish letters from various parts of the country describing the outdoor life and the opportunities for pleasure and for work these parts offer.[21]

This became the sanatorium patient's national magazine. It contained scientific articles and health information geared to the patient's level of understanding; poetry, articles, and letters written by patients; advertisements promoting the latest tuberculosis related fads; and a variety of maxims and proverbs that educated readers about the cure. Entries were often educational, sometimes humorous, occasionally sad and moving, but always related in some way to tuberculosis. The journal helped to expand the patients' world from the microcosm of the tiny porch on which they cured to the whole world arena of those similarly afflicted. The *Journal of the Outdoor Life* nourished their minds and spirits and, indirectly, challenged patients to make a literary contribution. It became, therefore, another important form of both education and therapy.

The D. Ogden Mills Training School for Nurses

By 1912 both Dr. Trudeau and Dr. Brown felt that the time had come to start a training school for nurses on the grounds of the sanatorium.

> *It is a well known fact that patients who have taken the cure of pulmonary tuberculosis, and who have any natural ability for nursing, are far better nurses for tuberculosis patients than some trained nurses without knowledge of tuberculosis. If to such women good training could be given in a two year course, we felt that a great need would be filled—many well educated girls, often college graduates, cured of tuberculosis could, after such training, follow useful lives, and many patients and institutions could be supplied with nurses who knew the modern treatment of pulmonary tuberculosis.* [22]

Trudeau School of Tuberculosis

Many years prior to his death, Dr. Trudeau was interested in starting a school that would provide physicians with a laboratory and clinical site for the purpose of broadening their tuberculosis education. Due to a lack of funds, this was one of the few dreams he had that was not realized until after his death. Prior to the establishment of this school, every opportunity was made for the young physicians who were patients at the sanatorium to use the Saranac Laboratory as well as the sanatorium laboratory for research work. In fact, most of the laboratory work that was performed in the area was conducted by curing physicians who were considered healthy enough to resume a limited work schedule. Ultimately, in 1916, the Trudeau School of Tuberculosis was formed and became a nationally known tuberculosis consortium that included the sanatoria, hospitals, and laboratories in

Saranac Lake and the surrounding areas. Instruction was given by the medical staffs of the participating institutions as well as by special lecturers who were brought in from New York City.

The goals of the school were to promote more interest in the disease as a medical specialty and also to give impetus to earlier diagnosis. It was also hoped that those attending the school would develop a more favorable attitude in relation to disease management and treatment. Furthermore, the school served as a clinical site for physicians or medical students desiring to gain

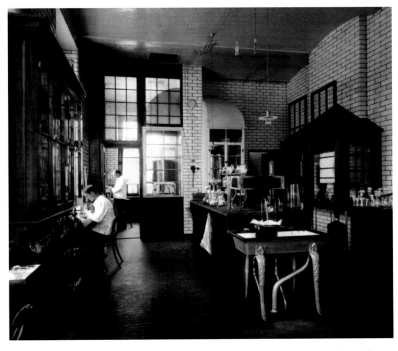

Student conducting research in the Saranac Laboratory in the village
Courtesy of the Trudeau Institute Archives

Ad for Trudeau School of Tuberculosis
"Journal of the Outdoor Life"

administrative experience in the organizational and managerial aspects of running a sanatorium. The public health work in the control of tuberculosis that was being actively pursued in Saranac Lake offered another focus of interest for the physicians attending the school. Although the courses were limited to a few weeks each year, there were additional provisions made for a limited number of students who wished to conduct research or study special problems related to tuberculosis.

The first six-week course was held on May 17, 1916, at the cost of $150 to $200. This fee included instruction, and room and board.

> No more fitting or better-equipped center for such a school could be found in the United States. Here, where Dr. Trudeau achieved his greatest success, will be opened an institution of learning that will do much to extend to every part of America the scientific and personal influence of the Great Pioneer.[23]

Prevention

Dr. Hermann Biggs, the New York State Health Commissioner, became the first to initiate a public health campaign directed against the spread of tuberculosis. In 1889 he sent a report to the Board of Health urging the city government to undertake a planned campaign against the disease. The report stressed that the disease was communicable and, therefore, careful collection and disinfection of infected sputum was imperative as was meticulous disinfection of every patient's inhabited surrounding. A few years later, in 1892, Dr. Lawrence Flick of Philadelphia spearheaded the formation of the first voluntary society, the Pennsylvania Society for the Prevention of Tuberculosis. This became the first organization that was formed specifically for the purpose of preventing tuberculosis. It remained the only voluntary organization in the battle against tuberculosis for eight years until a number of other state and local organizations began to develop.

As each of these organizations had a different agenda and list of individual priorities, for the sake of continuity, it was decided to establish a national tuberculosis organization in 1904. As a result, the National Association for the Study and Prevention of Tuberculosis (NASPT) was formed. Dr. Edward L. Trudeau was selected to sit as its first president. At the first annual meeting of the NASPT, Dr. Trudeau stressed the importance of education:

> The first and greatest need is education, education of the people and through them education of the state. It is evident that if every man and woman in the United States were familiar with the main facts relating to the manner in which tuberculosis is communicated and the simple measures necessary for their protection, not only might we reasonably expect as a direct result

of this knowledge a great diminution in the death-rate of the disease, but the people would soon demand and easily obtain effective legislation for its prevention and control.[24]

It was becoming increasingly obvious that not only did prevention have a significant impact on decreasing both the incidence and mortality rate of tuberculosis, but also that the sanatorium offered the best chance for a cure. The sanatorium, as an educational institution, thus became the ideal place to educate the patients in hygiene and sanitation. One of the first rules of instruction at the sanatorium was "Prevention of Infection in Others." It was believed that "if every discharged patient doesn't save three sound people by what he can teach them he wasn't worth saving."[25]

Shortly after Dr. Brown arrived at the sanatorium, he wrote a little book entitled *Rules for Recovery from Tuberculosis*, which was given to every patient upon admission. The content of the book covered every possible aspect of the disease with a major emphasis on prevention; specifically the care of sputum, disinfection, and cleaning. In the preface, Dr. Brown stated:

> *This little book has been written to help patients avoid blunders, which are very easily made at first, but very apparent to any patient who knows the problem. . . . It is not the author's intention that the book should be hastily read and laid aside, like the modern novel, but he believes that it should be read slowly, chapter by chapter, day by day. When it has been carefully read in this manner, he hopes it will be used as a book of reference, a handbook, so to speak, of the fundamental principles of cure.*[26]

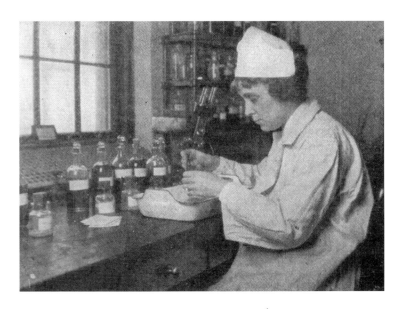

Nurse testing a patient's sputum at the sanatorium
Courtesy of the Trudeau Institute Archives

Sputum was to tuberculosis as blood is to AIDS. As sputum was the primary vehicle through which the disease was spread, there was nearly obsessive emphasis on its proper care. Any patients who violated sputum precautions were immediately discharged from the Trudeau Sanatorium. The care of sputum became such a topic of universal interest that the *Journal of the Outdoor Life* contained many advertisements that offered the latest fashions in individual sputum flasks. Dr. Brown wrote:

> *The care of the sputum should be above criticism, and the slightest infringement of rules about the sputum should be followed by summary dismissal. The sputum should all be burned and spitting into closets or lavatory-bowls must be guarded against. . . . Individual sputum cups should be provided and no general sputum boxes or cuspidors be allowed. . . . The clothing of many patients should be disinfected on arrival and it is a wise plan so to treat the clothes of all patients. . . . In a study of the dust from the cottages of the Adirondack Cottage Sanitarium only one specimen was found to contain "tubercle bacilli" and in this cottage a patient had been reported for carelessness.[27]*

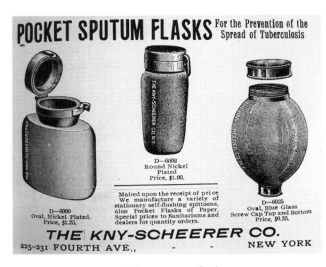

Ad for sputum flasks
"Journal of the Outdoor Life"

Despite the large tuberculous population, it was often reported that the chances of infection were much greater on a New York City subway than on the streets of Saranac Lake. Both the morbidity and mortality rates among the natives were far below what would normally have been seen in a population of a similar size. Those impressive rates gave testimony to the efficacy of the village campaign on education and prevention; the townspeople knew how it was transmitted and were fined if they disobeyed the ordinances that were directed towards dangerous behavior. For example, anyone caught spitting in a public place was fined fifty dollars.

Dr. Brown and others founded the Saranac Lake Society for the Control of Tuberculosis in 1907. Known as the T.B. Society, it was organized to control the disease of tuberculosis by:

Educating the people in regard to the proper sanitary measures in relation to tuberculosis by lectures, the distribution of literature, and other appropriate means.

Aiding the Board of Health in bringing home to the people the necessity of enforcing these measures, especially such as deal with expectoration and disinfection.

Encouraging and assisting all hotels and boarding houses to enforce these measures.

Maintaining a Free Bureau of Information for health-seekers.

To educate with a twist of humor, one patient wrote the following in the *Journal of Outdoor Life*:

The Adventures of T.B. Germ as Told by Himself

We are a large and varied family. I am of the Tubercular branch and my nearest and dearest relative, in fact my cousin, is the Pneumonia germ. Very fond of him I am, so fond in fact that wherever he chances to be I do my best to follow.

When first I awakened to the fact of my existence, I perceived myself in a dark dusty corner which was very cozy, I assure you. Not for long, though was I to stay there, for one day a woman came with a big thing called a Broom, and I was whirled into the air and the next thing I knew I had been swallowed by a Man. Down a dark passage I went, and then, lo, I beheld the most wonderful sight. I saw a great many little rooms and immediately I settled in one of these quite content. . . . But one fatal day the Man went on a Street Car, and although there was a sign, "Spitting Prohibited by City Ordinance," he wasn't overbright nor thoughtful nor cleanly, and so I soon found myself on the floor. All day I rode in the car, and the next morning another awful Broom came along and whirled me into the air, and for a moment I thought I was going out of the door into the fresh air and sunshine, and that would have been my death. With an effort I managed to cling to something in a crevice near a seat and when the door opened and another man came in I was lifted by a gust of wind right into his mouth.

Now this man was not careless and slovenly, and the minute I went down that dark passage I was sorry and continued to fret for a long time. I just could not seem to feel contented. One day I heard a noise like a thunder above me and the first thing I knew I was in a thing that was dark and awful and is called a Sputum Cup. Then I was taken to a place called a Laboratory. I was left there in that sealed box, while some one looked over the contents of the cup with a monstrous glass eye and found me and put me in an air-tight jar. Now I don't know how long I still have to live, but I don't believe it is long.

How I do wish that I had not had such an adventurous spirit! I might still be living comfortably in the careless Man's chest.[28]

Campus Life

The majority of patients at the sanatorium were young. At the turn of the last century, tuberculosis was responsible for more than one-third of all deaths between the ages of fifteen and thirty-five. Therefore, the highest percentage of consumptives at the Trudeau Sanatorium was between the ages of eighteen and thirty-five. Phil Gallos offered a wonderfully descriptive portrait of the young consumptive in his book *Cure Cottages of Saranac Lake*:

> They brought with them to Saranac Lake a lust for life and a resilience of spirit that, if anything, was enhanced and matured by the sobering realization that death was always so near. This combination of powerful opposites—youth and death—could ennoble the rude, inspire the apathetic, make wise the foolhardy, and ignite a desire in the most facetious to strip away all pretenses. The faces of some of these young patients expressed passion, courage, and an uncompromising frankness that was nothing short of awesome.

> Finally, the seriousness of the disease and the character of the cure forced all but the most unreflective patients into a fundamental confrontation with their goals, their values, and their innermost selves. Many emerged from the cure with totally reoriented systems of beliefs and priorities. They truly became different people; and they were glad, because they knew their exile to the "city of the sick" had given them an existential understanding of all those universal truths to which most people, caught up in the superficial minutiae of the day-to-day round, merely pay habitual lip service. For almost everyone who survived it, tuberculosis was a profoundly transformative experience; and they believed, far more often than not, that they were much the better for it. Considering all this, it does not seem so strange that many ex-patients regarded (and still regard) their curing days as the fullest, happiest, and most meaningful of their lives.[29]

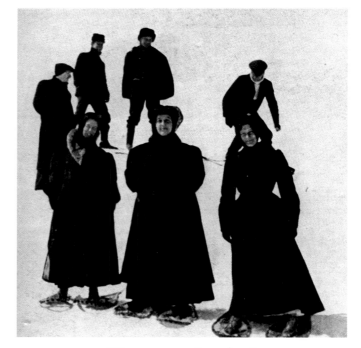

"Happiness on Snowshoes"
"Journal of the Outdoor Life"

Who these patients were had a major influence not only on the development of the Trudeau Sanatorium into a major educational center, but also on the tenor of life that gradually evolved both at the sanatorium and in the village. Out of a total of 6,513 patients discharged up to November 1924, there were 476 nurses; 371 physicians and medical students; 1,240 schoolteachers, students, lawyers, clergymen, dentists, architects, and engineers; and 1,418 clerks, stenographers, and book-keepers. They came from all over the world. Countless numbers of them stayed on and contributed their various talents to enhance the growth and development of Saranac Lake. Many were young and reckless, always willing to try the latest health related experiment. The sanatorium was a good proving ground for scientifically controlled treatments. After successful animal experimentation, a variety of new remedies were tried out on patients who were begging "to try anything the most Harebrained theorist might propose."[30]

DORMITORY LIFE Upon arrival at the sanatorium, the patients were admitted to the Reception Cottage where they remained for at least twenty-four hours. Here, they were closely observed and given a complete physical assessment. Their rooming assignment depended upon the severity of the disease. The more acute patients were assigned to an infirmary and put on complete bed rest.

> *Much thought and expense have been devoted to making [Childs Memorial Infirmary] at once homelike and practical. The interior is charmingly arranged. Outside there is a broad veranda surrounding three sides of the building with a Dutch door to each room through which the patients' beds may be conveniently rolled in and out. The view from the veranda is particularly fine and "Whiteface," the highest mountain in this region is an endless pleasure, reflecting as it does the ever-varying sunsets.*

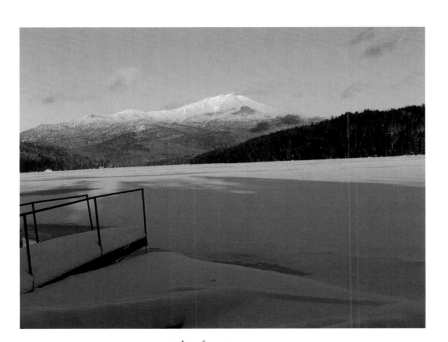

Whiteface Mountain
Photograph by Victoria E. Rinehart

The patients are expected to begin the "cure" at nine o'clock in the morning; at a quarter of one there is an intermission for dinner until two o'clock. [From two until four rest is required outdoors in a reclining position. Reading but no talking is allowed.] Very enthusiastic patients spend the evenings in the open air, beside sleeping out at night. These persons deserve to be cured. In the warm weather there is no excuse for not wanting to live out of doors, but in winter, in the severe cold, one is apt to regard this as a very cruel world and long for an excuse to go inside.[31]

Those with less severe symptoms were assigned to a cottage with patients of the same gender who were in a similar state of disease. As their conditions improved, they were progressively moved from cottage to cottage each prescribing the next incremental level of exercise and freedom. This created a homogeneous healing and social environment for the patients.

One patient wrote:

We were with people who were in the same boat, more or less. We didn't have some dying over here and feeling miserable and others running around over there and having a good time. I was in one of the cottages right away. They had a place where they admitted everybody and I was there for a day or two until they evaluated me to see where to put me. But they put me right out into a cottage. They started out our activities very slowly. For instance, we would start one meal a day going to the dining room. The other two would be delivered to the cottage. Then we would increase to two meals a day in the dining room and so on. After the third meal they would give us a fifteen-minute exercise. We could walk for fifteen minutes a day, then it would increase to thirty minutes once a day, then twice a day. That's the way they got us back on our feet.[32]

Another patient described her own progress:

I was at Ludington Infirmary, and then when I was one step better, I would go to a cottage where I wasn't allowed any exercise

Prescription for exercise
Courtesy of Anne Irene Remis

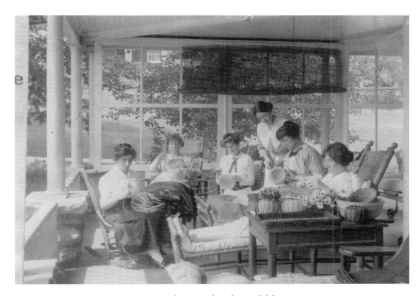

Curing on the porch of Penfold Cottage
Courtesy of the Trudeau Institute Archives

yet, and then to a cottage where I could be up a little bit. But we were mostly in bed, and all the meals came to us. And we had such a good time; it was so special. We developed such close relationships with our roommates. There was no TV, but we could read, we could write letters, and we could just be together. We would be on the porch all day in a bed. From there we went to an "up cottage" where there was more freedom.[33]

Other patients described their recollections of curing on the verandas during the colder months:

Many of the cottages have been built by friends, frequently as memorials, and bear the name of the donor. They consist usually of four separate bed rooms, a sitting room and bath, the chief feature of each being the large covered verandas furnished with comfortable chairs and cots and enclosed with glass at one or two sides to protect the patients from draughts while "taking the cure." It is here you find the patients from morning until late at night. However when the thermometer registers twenty to thirty degrees below zero, some vigilance is required to find them, for a figure carefully wrapped in rugs, with cap well pulled down, has proved to be a pillow with a newspaper pinned to the cuffs of the fur coat, while its owner was cuddled close to the fire inside the cottage![34]

Porch teas are customary afternoon dissipation and . . . summer or winter, may be seen groups of men and girls enjoying this mild form of excitement. In winter it is sometimes difficult to serve the tea hot, but excuses are unnecessary as all understand the penalty of staying in the house during the hours of "cure."[35]

Dr. Brown detailed a daily schedule that was "not to be blindly followed, but to serve as a basis for a talk with the patient's physician who alone is in a position to order most successfully the patient's time":

7:30	Awake. Take temperature.
	Milk (hot if desired) if necessary.
	Warm water for washing. Cold sponge.
8:00	Breakfast
8:30	Out of doors in chair or bed
10:30	Lunch when ordered
11 - 1	Exercise or rest as ordered
1 - 2	Dinner
2 - 4	Rest in reclining position. Reading but no talking allowed.
3:30	Lunch when ordered
4:00	Exercise in prescribed amount
6:00	Supper
7:00	Out on good nights
8:00	Take temperature
9:00	Lunch and bed. Once or twice a week a hot bath, followed by cold sponge.[36]

(Exercise means walking. Special permission must be obtained before indulging in other forms of exercise.)
None for one week, then ask about it.
None if feverish.
None if blood in sputum.
None if loss of weight.
None if fast pulse.
Never get out of breath.
Never get tired.
Never run.
Never lift heavy weights.
No mountain climbing.
GO SLOW.
Exercise regularly and systematically, whether rain or shine.
Walk up hill at start, so as to come down hill on return.
Remember always that you will have to return.
Rest one-half hour before and after meals.

Rules for Exercise
Courtesy of Anne Irene Remis

The childlike routine imposed on the patients was often a comfort. To many it made the days seem shorter. To others it restored some semblance of order to the chaos that the disease had wreaked upon their lives.

It was difficult, if not impossible, to separate out the curing activities from the activities of daily living. They became one and the same. Furthermore, the trilogy of rest, food, and air became almost a daily mantra.

According to Dr. Brown:

There are three great medicines in the treatment of tuberculosis; medicines which when rightly used are far superior to those found in any pharmacopoeia: rest, food, and fresh air.

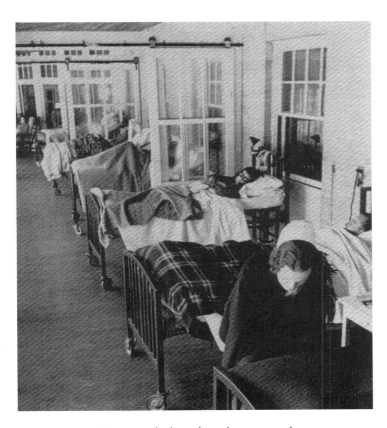

Curing in bed on the infirmary porch
Alfred Eisenstadt/TimePix

Rest allows the body to encapsulate the bacilli in the lungs, to wall off the spots of disease and to dam their poisons. . . . The excessive demands upon the body in tuberculosis has led to excessive waste of body substance and given rise to the popular name "consumption." The conservation of body substance is obtained through rest.

Good food, spiced with laughter, eaten with contentment, digested at ease, turns sour visages into sweet, bad health into good. Food not only supplies fuel and oil, but repairs the parts injured in the wear and tear of life. . . . The rule for the man underweight should be to eat as little food as he can in order to gain weight. . . . Three good meals a day, two or three glasses of milk, one or two eggs a day, cooked or raw, are often sufficient to add enough to his weight to bring him the gain he wished for. . . . The kitchen is the only pharmacy that many patients should know.

Fresh air is the best medicine! Two miles of oxygen three times a day. This is not only the best, but cheap and pleasant to take. It suits all ages and constitutions. It is patented by Infinite Wisdom, sealed with a signet divine. It cures cold feet, hot heads, pale faces, feeble lungs, and bad tempers. . . . Spurious compounds are found in large towns; but get into the country lanes, among green fields, or on the mountain top, and you have it in perfection as prepared in the great laboratory of Nature.[37]

The need for rest, food, and fresh air created an entire industry devoted toward those curing from tuberculosis. All kinds of devices such as sitting out chairs, windshields, bookcases for the porch, window tents, and sunlight enhancers were developed, marketed, and sold. Fur coats became a survival rather than a luxury item. Dairy farms dotted the landscape surrounding Saranac Lake.

Dr. Brown designed the Adirondack Recliner fashioned after a chair developed by Dr. Peter Dettweiler who cured in Dr. Brehmer's sanatorium in Germany. Dr. Dettweiler, who found that he did not have enough strength to walk in the open air following his cure, developed a bed and chair combination that had a movable cushioned back. This enabled him to "take the air" in relative comfort.

Dr. Brown similarly believed that:

> *The chair in which the patient sits out should be the most comfortable in the house. No expense should be spared upon it, for here the patient must sit for many hours a day. A good chair should elevate the feet from the floor, have a movable back, move easily on castors from place to place, be strongly constructed and be provided with a good cushion, useful alike for comfort and warmth.*[38]

Dr. Brown's Adirondack Recliner was made in Saranac Lake and sold by A. Fortune & Company. Later there were several other local manufacturers of cure chairs, which distributed their product to all major sanatoriums throughout the world. And even though the cure chair concept was developed in Germany, the chair remained almost exclusively a Saranac Lake product.[39]

In the more traditional university setting, the term "dressing up to go out" perhaps elicits an image of a young female coed endlessly trying on outfit after outfit hoping to find just the right attire in the hopes of favorably impressing her new young man. At the University of

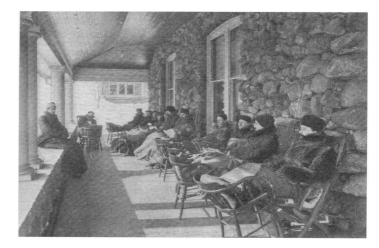

Curing before the advent of the Adirondack Recliner
Courtesy of the Trudeau Institute Archives

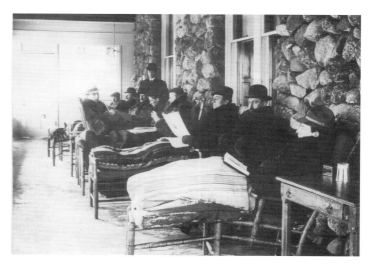

Curing after the advent of the Adirondack Recliner
Courtesy of the Trudeau Institute Archives

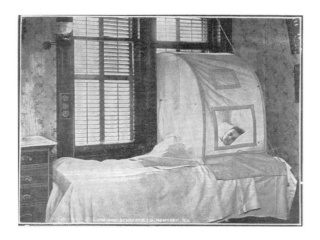

For those not able to go to a
sanatoriom, various types of
tents were available which
simulated an indoor, at home,
"outdoor" experience.

This ad illustrates just one of the
many types of home tents that
were available by mail order.
"Journal of the Outdoor Life"

Ad for locally manufactured recliners
"Journal of the Outdoor Life"

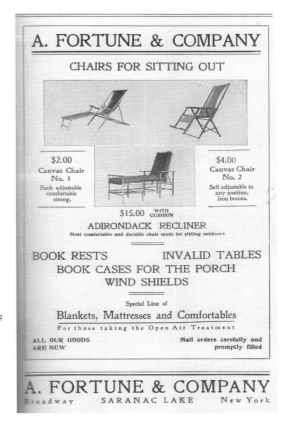

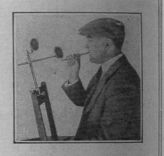

This device illustrates another do-
it-yourself treatment which
allegedly enhanced the healing
effect of sunlight. It allowed the
patient to self-direct the sunlight's
rays to a diseased portion of the
throat and larynx.
"Journal of the Outdoor Life"

Hope "dressing up to go out" had an entirely different connotation. It almost became a national pastime to discover the perfect combination of layered clothing that would protect the outdoor "curer" from the elements that often reached thirty to forty degrees below zero. Many who felt that they had arrived at a workable solution would publish their findings in the *Journal of the Outdoor Life*. For example:

> *Attire yourself in a long outing-flannel night-shirt, and over this put on another long woolen night-shirt, and over this a sleeveless sweater to protect your chest and shoulders. Put on your head one or two long-knitted skull-caps which can be pulled down to the end of your nose, and over your ears. Over these wear a knitted helmet which fits the head tightly, covers the neck, comes down over the shoulders, and leaves only the nose and mouth exposed to the open air. A hood knitted with Angora wool, of home manufacture, might take the place of the helmet.*

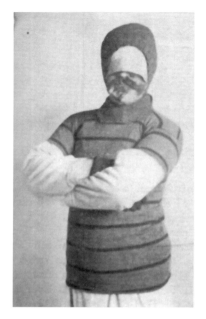

Dressing up to go out
"Journal of the Outdoor Life"

> *If necessary, a pair of cotton fleece-lined drawers and a pair of bed socks may be also worn; but in all ordinary winter temperatures they are unnecessary and would be uncomfortable. At first so much clothing will seem awkward and unpleasant; but one soon gets used to it; and when one wakes up in the morning feeling as if he had just returned from a delightful sleigh-ride, bright, fresh and enterprising, one is more than paid for any momentary discomfort.*

> *If one's nose grows cold when sleeping out, he is apt to nestle so far down in the bedclothes that he breathes the same air over and over again, thus defeating the very purpose of sleeping out. As a protection for the nose one sleeper-out we know of used, with satisfaction, a small piece of flannel, which was held in place by means of elastics slipped over the ears.*[40]

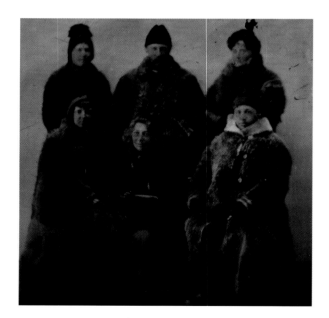

Patients keeping warm in 1896
Courtesy of the Trudeau Institute Archives

The patients who were up and about wore buffalo coats to keep warm. These were usually the general property of the sanatorium.

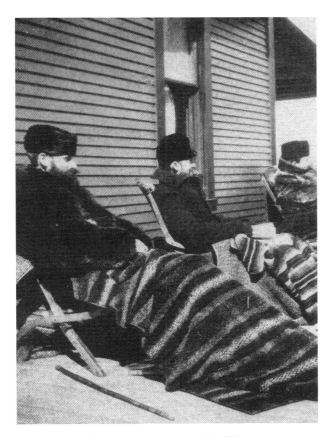

In addition to lap rugs and buffalo coats, beards were also a popular way for men to keep warm in 1893
Fritz Goro/TimePix

Dr. Brown felt it would be helpful to compile detailed instructions on how to wrap up in a cure chair. These directions were included in his little book, *Rules for Recovery From Tuberculosis*:

Place the rug, which should be large in size, fully extended on the chair. After sitting down grasp the part of the rug lying on the right of the chair and with a quick motion throw it over the feet and knees and tuck it well under the legs. Then do the same with the part of the rug on the other side of the chair but leave the edge free. Now grasp the free edge of the rug lying on the right hand side and pull it up and over hand until the end which was lying free beyond the feet is reached. Then pull up the far end of the rug, taking care to uncover as little as possible of the legs, and tuck both sides under the knees. This will give three or four layers of rug over most of the legs, but only one over the feet. It forms, however, a bag out of the rug and no air can enter. A second rug folded and thrown over the first makes such a covering that the coldest weather can be defied.[41]

As painful as sitting out on a porch in thirty degrees below zero could be, comparatively speaking, it was far from the most painful form of treatment used at the sanatorium. There were a variety of surgical techniques used, all of which attempted to rest the lung so that it could heal.

Many patients were subjected to a pneumothorax; often referred to by patients as a "pneumo" or "taking the air." Air was injected into the pleural cavity in order to collapse the lung, thereby enabling it to rest and heal. Once the air had been reabsorbed, the patients would return for periodic "refills" of air.

Two patients reminisced about their experiences with pnemothorax:

The first time I had a pneumo I thought I was going to die for sure. When I came out of it, whatever they gave me, I couldn't breathe, and I knew I was going to die, but I made it through the night. And the first month or so I would take it with local anesthetic. . . . Some of them never took any anesthetic, they just put the needle right in. The lung was completely collapsed; and it was amazing that it would come up again.[42]

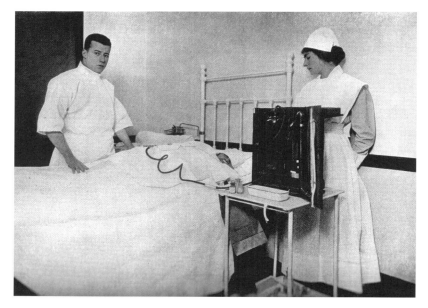

Patient receiving pneumothorax at Trudeau Sanatoriom in 1937
Courtesy of the Trudeau Institute Archives

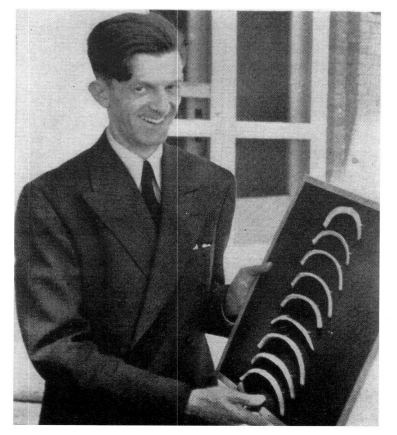

Patient who had nine ribs removed in 1937
Hansel Mieth/TimePix

I had to have pneumothorax continued for about seven years. It was very frightening, but it wasn't painful. It was scary but there was not real pain, because they anesthetized the area before they shot the big needle in. And the air was absorbed, and to prevent the lungs from re-expanding prematurely, they would replace the air every ten days to two weeks with two to seven liters [sic] of additional air.[43]

When rest, food, fresh air, and pneumothorax failed to bring about any significant improvement, the patient would often have to undergo a thoracoplasty. This was the most radical of therapies utilized and involved removing several ribs, causing that part of the chest wall to collapse upon the lung, thereby preventing any further respiratory movement. As the surgeons removed only the bone, leaving behind the periosteum, in time cartilaginous pseudo-ribs were generated which restored some level of support to the lungs. Because the surgery was so traumatic, it was usually done in stages. The surgical outcomes were questionable, however. Although the cure rate was reported to average thirty-five percent, the postoperative mortality rate ranged between ten to forty percent.[44] Later, this mutilating form of surgery was replaced by performing segmental resections or lobectomies (removal of a partial or complete lobe of the lung). This surgery resulted in a lower mortality rate and higher cure rate.

Many of the nurses talked of their recollections of the surgical care and thoracoplasties that were performed during the late forties and early fifties:

> When we had surgery at Trudeau Sanatorium we would be taken over to General Hospital. At that time there were a lot of TB doctors here and chest surgeons. Some of the best in the world were here because either they or a family member had come here to cure. Many would stay on and work here because they loved the area so much. We would pick our surgeon and he would take care of us. When it was time to leave the hospital we would go back to Trudeau. The surgeons would follow up with us at the sanatorium. All the doctors in town would come to a medical meeting once a week in the Recreation Hall where all the serious cases would be reviewed. There was excellent medical care for everybody—right across the whole spectrum.[45]

> At first they did thoracoplasties in often two and three stages. My husband had two or three. That was the most painful type of operation.[46]

> The thoracoplasties were awful. We could see people around town who had had them. They were all caved in and bent to one side.[47]

SOCIAL LIFE Care for the patients at Trudeau Sanatorium extended well beyond the meticulous attention that was given to the healing effects of rest, food, and air. In Trudeau's view, of nearly equal importance was the need to nurture the psychological well-being of the patients. The efficacy of his comprehensive holistic approach to patient care is not unlike the modern theories regarding the effects of stress on body systems; specifically the negative effect stress can have on the body's ability to resist infectious disease. Trudeau helped to ward off depression by actively involving all patients in some sort of occupational therapy program for the primary purpose of creating feelings of usefulness within each and every patient. He grouped together patients who were in similar stages of recovery in an attempt to prevent them from making unfavorable comparisons of different recovery rates. The many programs of health education assisted patients in guarding against overexertion, poor nutrition, and insufficient rest that could slow down recovery or precipitate a relapse of the disease. The social life that Trudeau cultivated at the University of Hope was another factor that contributed to the overall emotional well-being of the patients and was fondly remembered by all alumni long after they had graduated.

Perhaps one of the most important factors contributing to mental wellness was the spirit of optimism that was so fervently fostered by Trudeau. In a memorable presidential address before the Congress of American Physicians and Surgeons in 1910, Trudeau inspired physicians all over the world with his address on the *Value of Optimism in Medicine*. In speaking of the kind of optimism that "heals not only the sick body, but also the broken spirits of men as well" he stated:

> *Optimism is a product of a man's heart rather than of his head; of his emotions rather than of his reason. . . . Optimism is a prominent factor in anything a man may achieve in life. It is a mixture of faith and imagination, and from it springs the vision, which leads him from the beaten paths, urges him to effort when obstacles block the way, and carries him finally to achievement, where pessimism can see only failure ahead. Optimism means energy, hardships, and achievement; where pessimism means apathy, ease, and inaction. Optimism may, and often does, point to a road that is hard to travel, or to one that leads nowhere; but pessimism points to no road at all.*[48]

So much did Trudeau believe in the healing value of optimism, that in this world where illness reigned, patients were advised against discussing their symptoms with one another, as he believed that such a discussion could only serve to foster negativity and, thus, adversely affect the patient's mental process of healing. Optimism not only played a major role in the patients' perception of their recovery process, but also it seemed to pervade every aspect of their social life. Optimism, cheerfulness, and happiness, so much a part of life at Trudeau Sanatorium, were recurring themes that were alluded to over and over again by many recalling their years of curing.

The following passages offer a glimpse into that world of optimism as recalled by some of the patients:

The majority of us are apt to think of a Sanitarium for tuberculosis as having a depressing effect. I came here with something of a feeling that "who enters here leaves hope behind," but soon found my opinion erroneous; the patients are most cheerful and hope abounds. The absence of "talking of their ailments" is marked, except to allude to their trouble in a joking way the subject is seldom heard. All games of a violent character are forbidden; a good library, well equipped amusement pavilion and the pleasures the Adirondacks themselves furnish at all seasons, seem to suffice.[49]

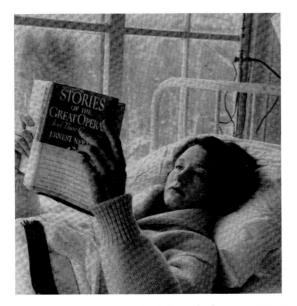

Keeping an active mind while on bed rest in 1937
Alfred Eisenstadt/TimePix

One is first impressed by the cheerful atmosphere of the place. . . . In the summer it is not difficult to imagine one's self at a summer hotel from which dancing and athletics have been excluded. After tea there is always someone at the piano and whether the music suits the taste of all or not, it induces conversation and lends an air of gayety. . . . The holidays of the year are observed with a variety of entertainment. Great preparations are made for Christmas. There is nothing lacking in the way of decorations and a great Christmas tree laden with gifts. If any one feels lonely or homesick, he keeps it to himself, so well is the spirit of Christmas observed. . . . All holidays each have their own appropriate celebrations. . . . In a collection of people as large as that found at the sanitarium, there are often several persons with unusual talents, which can be devoted to the pleasure of all. Music, acting, reciting, sleight of hand, are a few of the many ways of diverting the minds of the patients in the short evenings.

Even with all these amusements, the questions might be asked, "How do the patients worry through the long days and keep up a fair degree of cheerfulness?" Of those who spend their time in bed or who have the minimum of exercise, the answer might often be that the days are long and dreary. However, for them, if they will interest themselves in the great out-of-doors, there are the birds, plant and animal life to be seen, not to speak of the stars at night. The majority of patients, after a while, will give up useless regret and devote themselves to the "cure," at the same time agreeing with the old Italian saying "How sweet it is to do nothing."[50]

Happy is he who has simple tastes, who loves the flavor of the soil and can glean healthful pleasure from the changes of the seasons, the habits of the birds and insects, the secrets of nature, in short who can be content in watching the wonderful changes in the sky by day and by night. . . . The atmosphere is distinctly cheerful. Everywhere, lying in reclining chairs, on the porches are these rosy folk, some busy with sewing or reading, others are chatting cheerfully. If it is winter they seem entirely oblivious of the cold, but sit wrapped up in their rugs and fur coats with hot bricks at their feet and hot bottles in their laps, entirely comfortable, with snow or rain or what not a foot or two away. . . . Time does not drag to the wise patient who finds diversion in everything at his doorstep. The regular routine makes a day pass quickly. . . . Cheerfulness and hopefulness [seem] characteristic of this particular malady.[51]

If you will cast aside those dark glasses you have been wearing, and take a look at the sunrise or sunset, look at the reflection of the moon on the surface of Lake Flower, breathe in the air laden with the scent of balsam, pine spruce, and others of the evergreen family of trees, and get a view of the reflected sunset on the snow-clad slopes of Baker Mountain,—and, when you are "on exercise," take a walk down Bloomingdale Road in the dead of winter, with the snow crunching under foot, with every tree on the shores of the Saranac River creaking under the weight of beautiful white snow— if you can do these things and still say you have nothing to live for,—well I guess, then you haven't, and you might as well hang a "For Rent" sign between your eyes, north of your nose. . . . My experience has led me to judge that about the only pessimistic people in Saranac Lake are the people in good health who come here to visit their sick friends and relatives![52]

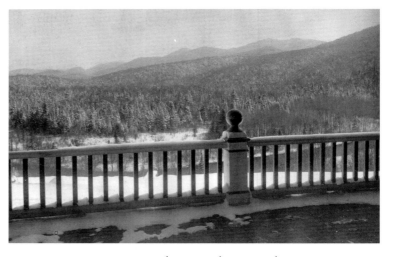
East view from McAlpin veranda
Courtesy of the Trudeau Institute Archives

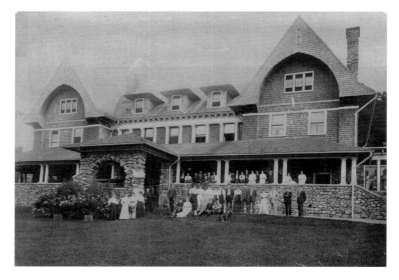
1899 Administration Building that contained the Dining Hall
Courtesy of the Trudeau Institute Archives

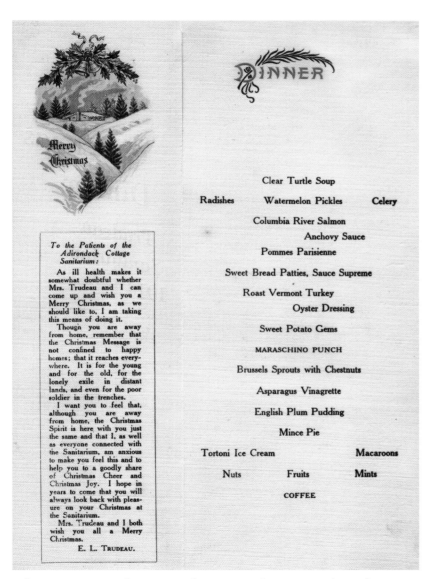

DINNER

Clear Turtle Soup

Radishes   Watermelon Pickles   Celery

Columbia River Salmon
Anchovy Sauce
Pommes Parisienne

Sweet Bread Patties, Sauce Supreme

Roast Vermont Turkey
Oyster Dressing

Sweet Potato Gems

MARASCHINO PUNCH

Brussels Sprouts with Chestnuts

Asparagus Vinagrette

English Plum Pudding

Mince Pie

Tortoni Ice Cream   Macaroons

Nuts   Fruits   Mints

COFFEE

To the Patients of the Adirondack Cottage Sanitarium:

As ill health makes it somewhat doubtful whether Mrs. Trudeau and I can come up and wish you a Merry Christmas, as we should like to, I am taking this means of doing it.

Though you are away from home, remember that the Christmas Message is not confined to happy homes; that it reaches everywhere. It is for the young and for the old, for the lonely exile in distant lands, and even for the poor soldier in the trenches.

I want you to feel that, although you are away from home, the Christmas Spirit is here with you just the same and that I, as well as everyone connected with the Sanitarium, am anxious to make you feel this and to help you to a goodly share of Christmas Cheer and Christmas Joy. I hope in years to come that you will always look back with pleasure on your Christmas at the Sanitarium.

Mrs. Trudeau and I both wish you all a Merry Christmas.

E. L. TRUDEAU.

Christmas menu with message of inspiration from Dr. Trudeau who was too ill to make a personal appearance
Courtesy of the Trudeau Institute Archives

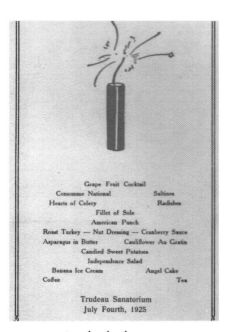

Grape Fruit Cocktail
Consomme National   Saltines
Hearts of Celery   Radishes
Fillet of Sole
American Punch
Roast Turkey — Nut Dressing — Cranberry Sauce
Asparagus in Butter   Cauliflower Au Gratin
Candied Sweet Potatoes
Independence Salad
Banana Ice Cream   Angel Cake
Coffee   Tea

Trudeau Sanatorium
July Fourth, 1925

Fourth of July menu
Courtesy of the Trudeau Institute Archives

Although food was considered a form of treatment, the process of eating was considered a major part of the social life. All the "up patients" would "dress" for meals and meander across the beautiful campus to the big dining room where they would take their nourishment. The tables were set with colorful tablecloths, sparkling crystal glasses, and shining silverware. On each patient's plate was a colorful menu, printed on the grounds, listing the current choice of entrées. In the background could often be heard someone playing classical music on a piano located in one of the nearby lounges. After the evening meal, patients would gather about the porch and make their social plans for the evening.

As remote as Saranac Lake and Trudeau Sanatorium were, the social and cultural opportunities for the patients often rivaled major metropolitan areas. Patients who were well enough to have town privileges could enjoy dining and movies in Saranac Lake; the village openly accepted consumptives as visiting residents of their village. There were picnics, parades, sleigh rides, plays from Broadway, and symphonies brought in from New York City and Boston.

A patient recalling a memorable sleigh ride in the early 1900s wrote:

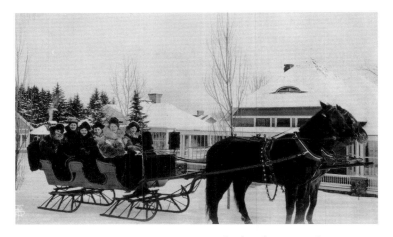

Patients enjoying a winter sleigh ride in 1906
Courtesy of the Trudeau Institute Archives

> *It took us an hour to prepare for the daily sleigh ride that was prescribed for everyone. We wore muffs, veils, mittens, huge galoshes, and buffalo robes and coats that were part of the sanatorium equipment. Hot bricks kept our feet warm. In the spring when the snow began to melt, we noticed black stumps along the sides of the road at regular intervals. Sometimes they ran across the road. Having come from Philadelphia, we were unaware of the rigors of an Adirondack winter and were amazed to learn that the stumps were the tops of fence posts!*[53]

There was the annual Winter Carnival which featured an illuminated ice palace constructed from blocks of ice painstakingly cut from the lake. For those confined to the grounds, there were costume balls, plays, and recitals given by patients; Sinfonietta performances that were brought in from the neighboring Lake Placid Club; and graduation exercises held for the patients who were being discharged.

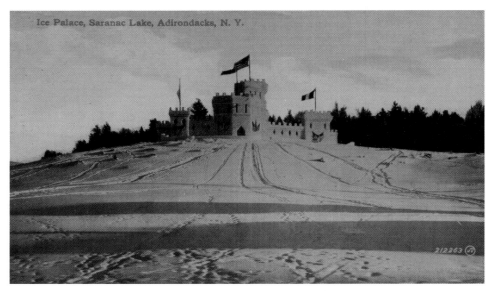

The Ice Palace at the Winter Carnival, Saranac Lake, NY
From the postcard collection of Florence H. Wright

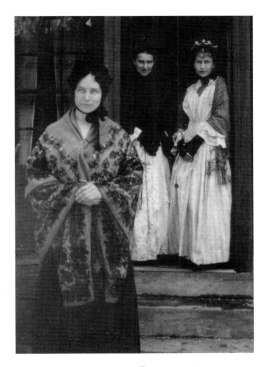

Costume Ball in 1925
Courtesy of the Trudeau Institute Archives

On February 20, 1925, the patients at Trudeau Sanatorium celebrated its fortieth anniversary. In honor of the anniversary, the patients held a costume ball depicting the period of 1885 when Dr. Trudeau started the sanatorium. Local residents of Saranac Lake helped the patients to get the proper clothes. Prizes were awarded for the best costumes.

The dinner tables were elaborately decorated and the superintendent of nurses awarded the prize for the best-dressed table. Dr. Francis B. Trudeau was the toastmaster and kept the guests entertained throughout the festive event. Patients told humorous stories about forty years earlier when those who came to die remained to enjoy renewed life and all that it offered.[54]

Music was seen as "Refreshment for the Sick." The concert noted in the accompanying illustration was brought to the sanatorium courtesy of the Lake Placid Club.

All patients at Trudeau Sanatorium were members of the Thursday Evening Club, which sponsored social activities, holiday parties, and other special events at the hospital.

Medical staff, nursing staff, local talent from surrounding areas, and sanatorium patients all

Melville Dewey, founder of the Dewey Decimal Classification System, was also the founding father of the Lake Placid Club in Lake Placid, New York. One of his many interests was simplified English spelling. In keeping with the nineteenth century efficiency movement, Dewey believed that English should be spelled phonetically to shorten reading and writing times. Dewey's work left its mark on the Lake Placid area where Adirondack Lodge is still called Adirondak Loj.

The program depicted in this picture reflects the simplified spelling advocated by Dewey.

A sentence written in Dewey's simplified spelling might read:

Speling Skolars agree that we hav the most unsyentifik, unskilarli, illojikal and wasteful speling ani languaj ever ataind.

Complimentary concert

by

Boston Simfony ensemble

at

Trudeau sanatorium

Wednesday 19 August 1925 at 3.15 p. m.

Orkestra

Daniel Kuntz, conductor

Julius Theodorowicz, violin	Gaston Bladet, flute
Frederick Sigl, violin	Louis Speyer, oboe
Vincent Mariotti, violin	Albert Ritter, timpani
Louis Artières, viola	Henri Girard, bass
Hans Pick, cello	Walter Hansen, piano

1 Lyric suite — Grieg
  a Shepherd's boy b Norwegian rustic march
  c Notturno d March of the dwarfs
2 Kamennoi-Ostrow — Rubinstein
3 Carmen : selection — Bizet
4 a Sonata pathétique : adagio — Beethoven
  b Marcietta — Sudessi
5 Jolly Vienna : waltz — Komzak
6 Babes in Toyland : selection — Herbert

Strict silence during music is Club custom
Please do not enter or leav during selection

Complimentary Concert in 1925
Courtesy of the Trudeau Institute Archives

contributed their talents to various social events. A 1925 program included a mouth organ recital; a medley of Scotch airs; a presentation of x-ray plates; a recitation contest, including *Symptoms* and *My Fibrosis*; a violin concert; and a hypnotism demonstration. A local high school drama director offered a humorous drama presentation, and two nurses entertained by playing the piano and singing.

Indigenous to college social life is use and misuse of alcohol. It was no different at the University of Hope. Alcohol at the sanatorium, although forbidden, could be found hidden away in many of the cottages. Saranac Lake, in the 1920s, enjoyed a very active bootlegging business with liquor smuggled down from the nearby Canadian border.

> *Drugstores sold alcohol in nursing bottles, and a dry-cleaner tucked pints into the pockets of garments returned to the customer. The serpentine "Rum Trail" ran from Champlain near the border to Glens Falls, Saratoga, and Albany. . . . Rumrunners dodged through the mountains and reached Saranac on the dirt roads of Franklin and Clinton counties. They used a convoy system, sending a pilot car ahead of the shipment. The scout car carried no contraband, and if the driver was detained that too warned the caravan.*[55]

In Dr. Brown's little *Rules for Recovery from Tuberculosis* book, he had the following to say regarding use of alcohol:

> *The value of alcohol in the treatment of tuberculosis is very slight, if any, and the danger from its use very great. . . . The experience of American sanatoriums, where almost without exception alcohol is prohibited under penalty of expulsion, bears ample evidence that it is not necessary as a stimulant and rarely as a drug. . . . Great danger lies in the fact that a man with nothing to do but to take "the cure" is very likely to go to excess when once he begins to use alcohol. If it gains hold upon him his only course is to cut loose from his boon companions and change his residence.*[56]

A graduate patient recounted the following story regarding his misuse of alcohol while at the sanatorium:

I was an ambulatory patient in the Phoenix Cottage. After our evening meal, a group of us took our walking exercises as prescribed, but instead of staying on the grounds we went to get some beer, which was totally against rules. There were about four of us in the little cottage, and we spent that evening having a grand time drinking beer and playing cards. And who walked in but the night supervisor of nursing, Miss Fitzpatrick. She was one tough nurse who said, "You broke the rules and are all going to suffer for this." We were quite afraid of her and we knew that if we violated the rules we could be sent home for misbehaving. We were all young boys, nineteen or so, who were very worried, as we didn't want our parents to know that we might be expelled from Trudeau for misbehaving. So we decided, as a group, to write a very eloquent letter to the doctor and try to argue or explain or plead our way out of the problem. We spent the rest of the evening composing the letter and, as luck would have it, I was designated to be the spokesman. When I got to his office the next morning he told me to sit down and read the letter to him. While I was reading, I noticed he had a very dour expression on his face. When I was finished, he waited for an interminable moment before saying, "All right; you can go back and tell your roommates that this time will be the last time it will ever happen." And let me tell you, it never happened again! We were so overjoyed at not being asked to leave that we felt like celebrating; although certainly not with beer! Imagine being so delighted at not being asked to leave a hospital. That should give an indication of how much we loved being there.[57]

Smoking was also a common pastime. Unlike alcohol, it was discouraged but not forbidden. For fire safety reasons, however, its use was restricted to the outdoors. Today it certainly seems ironic that smoking was allowed among patients trying to recover from lung disease. But in the early 1900s, little was known with scientific certainty about the deleterious effects of smoking on lung tissue. On smoking, Dr. Brown made the following comments:

As a matter of fact tobacco injures fewer men than excess in eating. On the other hand, the nicotine, the active principle of tobacco, is very poisonous when taken pure. One-tenth of a grain of nicotine will kill a dog in a few minutes. . . . Curiously enough the cause of the pleasure of smoking has not been determined and seems not to have been proved to be due to nicotine. It may possibly be due to the action

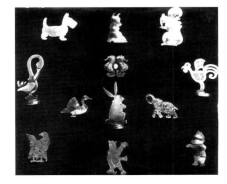

Sterling silver cigarette extinguishers made in the Trudeau Workshop
Courtesy of the Trudeau Institute Archives

of the smoke on the mouth, nose, and throat. Knowledge of its action upon a diseased lung is of considerable importance. Unfortunately little is known, though there is some evidence to show that rabbits when treated with small doses of nicotine combat disease less vigorously. . . . Moderate smoking then, for a healthy adult, who tolerates well the nicotine, seems to exert little harm.[58]

On any campus where young people are grouped together for an extended period, relationships are certain to flourish. Relationships that started on traditional college campuses were said to pale in comparison to those that often developed at Trudeau. Despite the unconditional acceptance of the consumptive population by the residents of Saranac Lake, the world from which the patients came was not always so accommodating. Some patients felt so stigmatized by their disease that when writing to friends at home they diverted their letters through a post office in Lake Placid or some other "acceptable" location in order to disguise the true origin of the correspondence. The world in which these people lived for so many months or years became, for many, a protected womb-like environment. There are numerous accounts of patients who, having demonstrated a full recovery, showed signs of relapse as their impending discharge date approached. For many, it was extremely difficult to reenter a world that had been vacated, in some cases, for years. Often the family that was left behind, in order to self protect, experienced what could be called anticipatory grieving. Assuming the worst, they grieved prematurely, and when the loved ones actually did return home, they were not always openly welcomed. This factor, coupled with the irrational fear of tuberculosis that was so prevalent, made reentry a difficult if not impossible task.

Although romances at Trudeau were strongly advised against, they flourished:

> *The practice became a sort of undergraduate ritual with its own argot: your lover was a "cousin," the affair itself was called "cousining," and the favorite trysting place on the Trudeau grounds, a small rest pavilion, was the "Cousinola."*[59]

Cousining developed mostly between patients, but occasionally between nurses and patients. Some cousins were already married to others on the outside, and others were single and ultimately married one another in the little chapel on the grounds of the sanatorium.

Two patients had the following to say regarding romance at the sanatorium:

There were flirtations and romances with the new crop of student nurses who arrived each six or eight weeks, and a patient population mainly young and often well educated. . . . We all looked better than anybody coming to visit us.[60]

After we get over the first shock of the idea of tuberculosis and are packed off to a community where, happily for us, we discover a great many people are going through the same thing, why we begin to respond, to recover. It's comforting. But when the time comes to step back into the other world again, it is no longer the problem of damage to lung tissue we have to battle, but the damage to our ego—sometimes irrevocable damage. All the girls are looking for some way in which to renew their faith in themselves. They react as any woman might who considers herself disfigured, deformed even. They lose confidence in themselves, and the result is so often just this—this constant need for reassurance. I'm amused with those Bright Things who tell [us] smirkingly: "But I thought people with pulmonary tuberculosis always had an inordinate sexual desire." Rubbish! More likely an inordinate need for love and affection. An inordinate desire, perhaps, to feel desirable.[61]

Although many patients spoke of the aphrodisiac effect of tuberculosis, none of the patients and nurses who were interviewed for this book could remember any patients becoming pregnant during the course of their cure. Bea Sprague Edward, a ninety-two-year-old graduate of Trudeau and nurse who worked at the sanatorium for several years, stated:

I don't recall that there ever was a pregnancy. I think part of the reason may have been medical. When the patients became ill, oftentimes they lost a great deal of weight and their menstrual periods stopped. Therefore becoming pregnant may not have been possible. In all the years I was there, I never heard of or suspected a pregnancy. It may also have been that very, very few of these cousining cases ever reached that stage. I think they were mostly just sort of smooching a little, spending time with one another, and going out for dinner together. Nothing ever happened that the staff heard about.

And please excuse me, but you will find that cousining is actually spelled cozening. If you look it up in the dictionary, you will find that cozening means, "to deceive, cheat, or defraud." That was the derivation of the word—one person cheated on another.[62]

Although all of the literature describing the tuberculosis era spells the word as "cousin," Bea Sprague Edward was spot on right! The dictionary does define "cozen" as one who deceives, cheats, or defrauds. Perhaps it would have been more accurate to use the term "cousining" to describe the romantic relationship that developed between unmarried patients, and limit the term "cozening" to only those relationships that developed between patients who were already married to others on the outside world.

The humorous poem that follows was written by a sanatorium patient and published in the *Journal of the Outdoor Life* in 1904.

"Cousins" Once, But, Etc.
Now I must admit right sadly
That once I loved quite madly
A captivating patient in the San,
So with beating heart I sought her,
And when alone I caught her,
I opened up my soul and thus began:—

"My Sweet, I love you dearly;
Distracted I am nearly
And my temperature is passing ninety-nine,
For I cannot live without you,
There's such a charm about you
And now my "cousin" love, will you be mine?"

Then I sat in silence waiting,
While my heart was palpitating
She looked so sweet, I nearly lost my head,
As her glorious eyes she lifted,
This girl so bright and gifted,
As she oped her ruby lips and softly said:—

"Purl two, knit two, right across the back;
Cable every thirteenth row—
There! You've thrown me off the track.
I've lost a count and dropped a stitch
Don't you know any better?

You shouldn't try to cousin a girl,
When she's knitting on a sweater."

Now I do not mind confessing,
That this was right depressing
When I thought she'd gently smile and answer "yes."
So I said: "Sweetheart, you're cruel;
And you are only adding fuel
To the flame of my devotion and distress."

Then she smiled and in her eyes
Was reflected from the skies
The blue of heaven itself from overhead;
And the sunlight bright and fair
Fell athwart her golden hair
Like a holy angels nimbus, as she said:—

"Knit two, purly two, just an inch and a half:
Cable every thirteenth row—
Now stop! Or you'll make me laugh;
For when you ask me for my hand,
What could I say more fit,
When you interrupt my knitting count,
Than just this one word—NIT."[63]

Alumni

Many who came to cure, recovered and graduated but, by choice, never left. Although they were free to return home, many elected to stay on seeking some form of employment on the grounds. Numerous others recovered, graduated, and left only to return, year after year, as alumni. It is almost impossible to conceive of a hospital in existence today that would engender that kind of reverence in its former patients. Admittedly, some stayed on out of fear of reentry due to the social stigma of the disease. But the greatest majority stayed on out of a love for all that the sanatorium offered: a healthy and mentally stimulating environment, and nearly unconditional acceptance.

As previously mentioned, the patient population comprised a wide assortment of occupational talent: physicians, nurses, teachers, architects, engineers, clerks, bookkeepers, etc. Many chose to stay on for no other reason than to give back to the place and people they considered their salvation. Ultimately, many of these people shaped not only the sanatorium but the little village of Saranac Lake as well. It was said by many that the best health care in the world could be found at Saranac Lake because internationally known physicians and surgeons came to either cure or be with a loved one who was curing. Furthermore, architects William Coulter, William Scopes, and Maurice Feustmann all came to Saranac Lake to cure. They stayed on to "draft some of the greatest of the Adirondack Great Camps, as Mr. Coulter did, and to become nationally respected specialists in sanatorium design, as did Messrs. Scopes and Feustmann."[63] Many of the young women that came to cure entered the nurse's training school and, when cured, stayed on to provide nursing care to others both on the grounds and in many of the cure cottages that had blossomed in the village.

During the summer months many patients who were considered cured returned as summer alumni. They returned year after year, checked back into the sanatorium for a month or two, and "replenished" their cure.

> For the most part patients would be at Trudeau for a couple of years at a time and it became one big happy family. And then when they went home, they were considered cured, but they would come back every summer and spend a couple of months or a couple of weeks. Everybody looked forward to friends coming back.[65]

In 1987, 1990, and again in 1993, Saranac Lake held a reunion for those who took the TB cure. A total of nearly 300 people returned from as far away as California for the three reunions. The reunions were held partly in an attempt to resurrect the history of the curing days at Saranac Lake, but also to provide a time of reminiscing with old graduates of the sanatoriums and cure cottages. The alumni ranged in age from sixty to ninety and all were able to keep up with the busy schedule planned for the reunion. Among the many activities were lectures on the current state of TB, as well as on AIDS in relation to its similarities in image and symptomology to TB. "It was all so emotional. There was such a sense of reminiscing, but there was also a thread of sadness that ran through as so many of these people lost friends here who were not cured."[66]

This little world of healing at Trudeau Sanatorium was not always utopian. There were some patients whose lives were delicately suspended by a gossamer thread that stretched tenuously between here and hereafter. They knew not when that thread would break. They marked time in seconds and minutes, rather than in days, months, and years. But that uncertainty did not stop one young patient from continuing to give until his "great heart that dared not beat too fast" slowed for the last time. He gave so that others in the sanatorium could receive. He gave for no other reason. One that wrote about his passing said, "This is the first and perhaps the last time that he of whom I write will be referred to in printed words." He was wrong.

This is the story of John Theodore Dalton, or Jack, as his friends called him. It is just one story about one patient who lived and died at Trudeau Sanatorium. There were most likely countless other "Jacks" who can never be remembered because their histories were lost or never recorded. What follows is not only a tribute to John Dalton, but also to all the "Jacks" and "Janes" whose life stories at Trudeau Sanatorium will forever remain unknown.

Jack, born in Vancouver, Washington on December 27, 1899, was a multitalented man who had charm, youth, good looks, high spirits, and tuberculosis. He attended the Iowa State College at Ames, Iowa. During the war he was a member of the Student Army Corps and, during the summer of 1918, he taught wireless telegraphy for the War Department at New York University. Later, in 1919 and 1920, he attended Dartmouth College in Hanover, New Hampshire where he was a member of Gamma Delta Epsilon. He entered England's Cambridge University in 1921 as a special student in the classics.

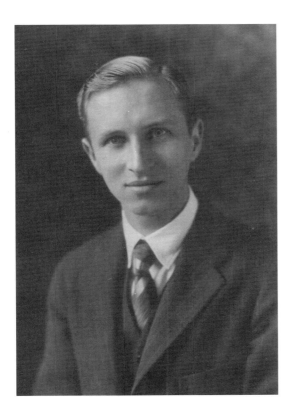

John Theodore Dalton, 1899-1927
Courtesy of the Trudeau Institute Archives

His illness was attributed to the influenza epidemic of 1918, from which he suffered and recovered, although never completely. On the eve of his graduation from Cambridge, he was stricken with tuberculosis. Saranac Lake remained his only hope.

The *Adirondack Daily Enterprise* offered the following information about Jack:

He was hopelessly ill from the time he came to Saranac Lake, but he gave without stint his time and such energy as he possessed to the development of ideas for making his fellow patients happier. He is credited with having brought the radio within reach of all patients in the Trudeau Sanatorium, those in the infirmaries as well as those in the cottages. He wrote and directed the production of a play, "Tom Tooney of Trudeau," which was presented by the Thursday Evening Club in December, 1925. He composed two songs, "Oh, Yes, Oh, No;" and "Land of Dreams," both of which were published and had some success. The latter was written while he was a patient in the Ludington Infirmary, too ill to be about the grounds. His charm and high spirit enlisted the friendship of many notable individuals, including Robert Hobart Davis, who wrote in his column, "Bob Davis Recalls" in the "New York Sun" a warm tribute to "A Great Heart that Dared Not Beat Too Fast." [The text from that article follows.] Many other well known literary, theatrical and musical men and women knew and loved Dalton and never missed an opportunity to call on him when they visited the Adirondacks.[67]

Shortly after Jack's death, his poems, written during his stay at the sanatorium, were rescued from the wastebasket and later published.

It might have been just as well had they not been rescued and printed. But the boy who wrote them was a brave and noble character. If this small volume will keep him a little longer in the memory of men and, perhaps, win a smile or draw a tear, the author and his verses will whisper a contented, "We thank you."[68]

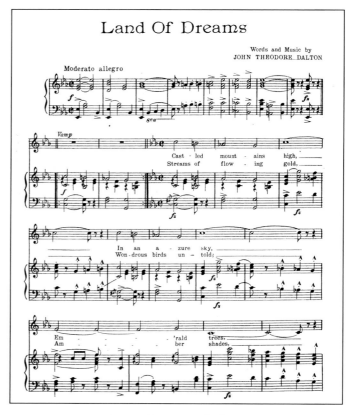

Partial score from "Land of Dreams"
Courtesy of the Trudeau Institute Archives

To those who know naught of the disquietudes of this life, to those who are strong in body and have not felt the afflictions of the flesh, to those who are unburdened by misery and feel naught of pain, this tale of fortitude is commended. For it is they who will pause in the midst of their contentment and wonder how one oppressed could go so far.

This is the first and perhaps the last time that he of whom I write will be referred to in printed words. No decorations will be conferred upon him, no public demonstration will mark his exit from a world through which he passed like a ray of warm light, touching mankind with benignant radiance. As I write these lines the aurora is fading.

Four years ago he took up his residence in those friendly mountains to face the great ordeal. But he had come too late. The inevitable could be postponed but not averted. Realizing that his tenure was brief, but desiring to make the span worthwhile, he went about the work of building a radio set that could be tuned in with the outside world. That cosmic touch through the ether aroused his interest and stimulated his imagination. He became adept with his homemade instruments, capturing the babble of distant cities, the music of new voices, the mirth and laughter flung on the wave lengths of the nation.

Into the hospital he brought the news of the hour, the orchestras of the gay places, the baseball scores, the story of the day's doings. For his afflicted and imprisoned companions he built other radio sets so that there came at nightfall to the high Adirondacks echoes from "home." With feverish haste he multiplied the implements of communication, consuming his vitality in perfecting the battery of contacts. Valiantly he fought the white plague with song and story.

During the last four years of his life he had faced the future with a tranquil heart, living only to bestow happiness upon his fellow sufferers. The pallor continued to creep upon him, revealing the cheekbones through its waxen field. Patients who were slightly touched came to the hospital in time, got cured, listened to his radios and went their way, blessing the pale trumpeter who mastered the dials. The rule that a patient could remain but one year was broken in his case and he stayed on, hopeless but uncomplaining, until the frail body surrendered. In his eyes still burned the flame of his indomitable will. Lying among his pillows he conducted the work of constructing his receiving sets. Two other patients, realizing the importance of continuing the labor he had begun, volunteered to carry on. He was like a dauntless leader stricken on the field, directing his lieutenants as the life tide ebbed.

Two weeks ago, when the World Series was on and the occupants of the Saranac retreat were clamoring for the news that was being flashed throughout the United States, the recumbent zealot laid his plans so that every pair of ears in the institution should hear the news for which they hungered. From the spells of lethargy and coma he roused himself and with intermittent whispers and fluttering gestures conducted the work of bringing the Big League to the bedsides of his flushed and expectant audience.

Despite his physical torpor he ruled the preparations with his spirit. With deliberate and painful motions he pointed out the way to still the static and enrich the tone. When the voices from the field began to come in clear and audible he sank back, a soft smile creeping over his ghostlike countenance.

An attendant, leaning over the wraith, prepared to adjust the head set to the sick man's ears. "We want you to hear," said he. "No," murmured the shadow. "It . . . would . . . make . . . my . . . heart . . . beat . . . too . . . fast. Tell . . . me . . . the . . . score . . . tomorrow."

Every other patient heard the results at the same instant it reached the ears of millions of American fans throughout the country, heard the cheers, the clamor at the stadium, the shouts of a mob gone mad and the aftermath.

The one man entitled to hear the reverberations that had penetrated the void and filled the air in the Saranac retreat dared not listen lest the wild ecstasy quicken the beating of his heart— lest that momentary exhilaration, that must-be-postponed happiness, send a gust of coughing through his tortured frame.

For those who had come to regard him as the link between them and the outer world he had staged the drama of the national game. At the supreme moment in the production the inspired director, satisfied to have brought happiness to those about him, closed his eyes in the restless sleep of pain.

"Tell . . . me . . . the . . . score . . . tomorrow." What score?
We weave the laurel for the brow of brawn, but none for fortitude.[69]

Land of Dreams

Castled mountains high
In an azure sky,
Emerald trees,
Lilac breeze.
Princess of this land,
Your hand
And heart I so much want to take,
But I might wake.

My land of dreams,
Why can't you be reality?
Just bright moon-beams,
And yet you mean so very much to me.
Dream one, play fair;
Just say you care,
And tell me where,
O'er fields and streams,
Your vision gleams,
Beyond my land of dreams.

Streams of flowing gold,
Wondrous birds untold;
Amber shades,
Twilit glades.
Prince of this strange land,
My hand
And heart I'd love to have you take;
I'm 'fraid we'd wake
~John Theodore Dalton

The Story of Anne: A Close-Up View

I arrived at Trudeau Sanatorium in 1939, at age twenty-three, and left for rehabilitation about ten years later. I had spent all but two years of this time in Ludington Infirmary as a bed patient. Hitler also arrived at this time in Czechoslovakia and proceeded as far as he could into Europe. Many people who fled from Prague, as members of the government cabinet of this country, later became "tenants" of Ludington Infirmary. They had fled on skis down the Alps into Italy; boarded a boat to China, and then later arrived at Trudeau. A Russian princess, several doctors from Havana, Cuba, and a daughter of a Norwegian Merchant Marine Captain were also in the infirmary and became good friends of mine. These interesting people made life friendly and comfortable. It was amazing how one could be so sick yet so happy. So near was joy to sorrow, yet it somehow blended to form happiness.

Time passed quietly and peacefully in prayer, study, and socialization. My occupational therapist was a beautiful woman who had two sons ready for college. Her husband had recently died leaving her with their sons to guide and educate. One day she mentioned that one son was confused and nervous as to whether or not to study medicine as his father had wished. She told him, "Ask your stomach for a decision!" He replied, "Is that where some people have their brains?"

I remember making a sterling silver baby spoon for my Godchild with my occupational therapist's help. It took months to make as I worked only minutes a day on it. First, I cut the handle from a slab of silver. Then I worked weeks on the hollowed out end for the bowl of the spoon. I insisted it had to be perfect and beautiful. Next, I wrote the child's name in cursive (Palmer method) penmanship on another slab of silver. Weeks later, with a jig saw, I

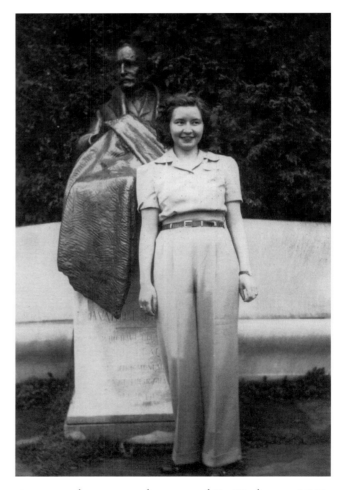

Anne standing next to the statue of Dr. Trudeau in 1941
Courtesy of Anne Irene Remis

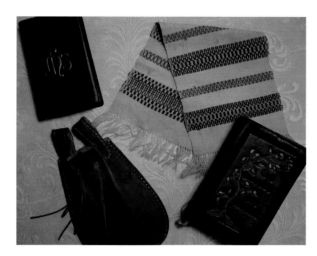

Articles made by Anne in occupational therapy
Courtesy of Anne Irene Remis

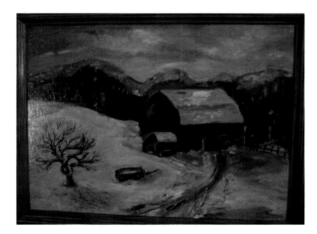

"Red Barn on Smith Road at Trudeau" with Mt. Baker and Old Saddleback in the background. Painted in 1947 by Anne Irene Remis.
Courtesy of Anne Irene Remis

started to saw his written name from the slab. It was satisfying work. Finally, I adhered his name carefully to the handle of the spoon, which was bent for easy grasping. After months of polishing, it was finally ready. I loved this little gem so much that I kept it by my bedside for viewing for a long time before I wrapped it up and posted it to my Godchild.

I waited anxiously for some glowing words that the gift had been received and loved. When no word came, I finally asked for an acknowledgement of the gift. Everyone was reluctant to tell me that the first time the little spoon had been used it was inadvertently dumped into the trash and lost forever. I was satisfied not sad. In the work there was pleasure of a skill learned and a gift given. I believed that I had stock in the landfill and that my shares held gems that paid the highest dividends.

My eight years of bed cure were busy. I managed to engage in leatherwork; tooling a small pocket book and two book jackets on which I painted titles and designs in color. The books are still in use today. A small lap loom was also brought to me in bed so that I could make doilies. There seemed to be no end to the activities and the time passed quickly.

My favorite craft was oil painting, but that was hard work for me since I did not possess an innate ability for painting. Skill took the place of artistic ability and, in 1947, I stopped painting after completing the "Red Barn on Smith Road at Trudeau." This was considered to be a "well done primitive painting" by the resident experts.

My other painting, the "Head of the Madonna," was termed "well done." The former painting was a result

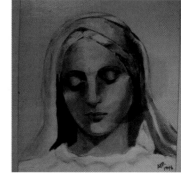

"Head of the Madonna" painted by Anne Irene Remis in 1946
Courtesy of Anne Irene Remis

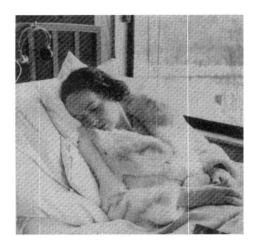

Trudeau veteran Isabel Smith had been bedridden ten years when "Life" photographed her here in 1954.
Fritz Goro/Timepix

of my being allowed my first fifteen minute prescription to walk after spending eight years in bed. I sketched the scene in charcoal in seven and a half minutes and carried the sketch back to bed in order to complete the painting.

At Trudeau we enjoyed private rooms throughout. Our beds were rolled out onto a porch of two rooms per patient. My porchmate was the incredible and unforgettable Isabel Smith. Izzy wrote her book, "Wish I Might," in 1955. [Isabel was a nurse who came to Saranac Lake in 1928 to cure and subsequently spent twenty years in bed. She was under the care of Dr. Francis B. Trudeau who ultimately gave her away in marriage in 1949, in the little chapel on the grounds of the sanatorium.] Our porch was touching the edge of Mt. Pisgah, making our view an all season moving and inspirational panorama.

I loved Trudeau. The doctors were superb. I remember once being given a prescription by my doctor for a correct shade of lipstick to match my pajamas! During my years at Trudeau, I underwent nearly every phase of tuberculosis therapy. Aside from bed rest, healthy food, and fresh air, (my initials, which spell AIR, took on a whole new significance for me), I also underwent almost every type of treatment for resting my lungs. When artificial pneumothorax failed to improve my condition, I was treated with phrenic nerve compression and later surgical severing of that nerve in an attempt to permanently collapse my lung. When that failed to offer me relief, I finally had to undergo a thoracoplasty in which several of my ribs were removed to prevent lung motion beneath the ribs. Today, when doctors view the scar at my neck from the

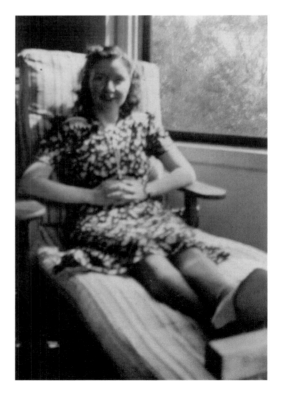

Anne reclining in her cure chair
Courtesy of Anne Irene Remis

severing of the phrenic nerve they often ask me if I had once attempted to slit my throat! Few doctors today are aware of all that we were put through, in the name of cure, those many years ago.

During the winter of 1940, safely tucked away in a Pullman car's upper berth, I experienced a sleepy and cold trip to New York City for medical treatment via the Adirondack Railroad. I left Saranac Lake in late evening scheduled to arrive at 6:30 a.m. the following morning at Grand Central Station in New York City where my brother was to meet me. He was there, but I was not. I had become a missing person!

Officials soon discovered that my Pullman car had been detached and abandoned on the tracks at Lake Clear Junction. The rest of the train had gone on without me. I was alone and completely unaware of the problem. I had spent the night as safe as a "bug in a rug" in my bed wearing my new muskrat fur coat. I had become so used to lying patiently in bed that it never occurred to me to question the lack of motion or silence. Those were the days of safety! I was delivered the following evening, twelve hours later, at Grand Central Station hugging my new fur coat and my brother.

I am now retired and have been gifted with an endowment of twenty-nine years in which I taught and researched children with cerebral palsy. At the age of eighty-six, I can still look back on my years at Trudeau as some of the happiest years of my life.

Written by Anne Irene Remis,
Clinton, New York, October 2001

Anne Irene Remis, October of 2001
Courtesy of Anne Remis

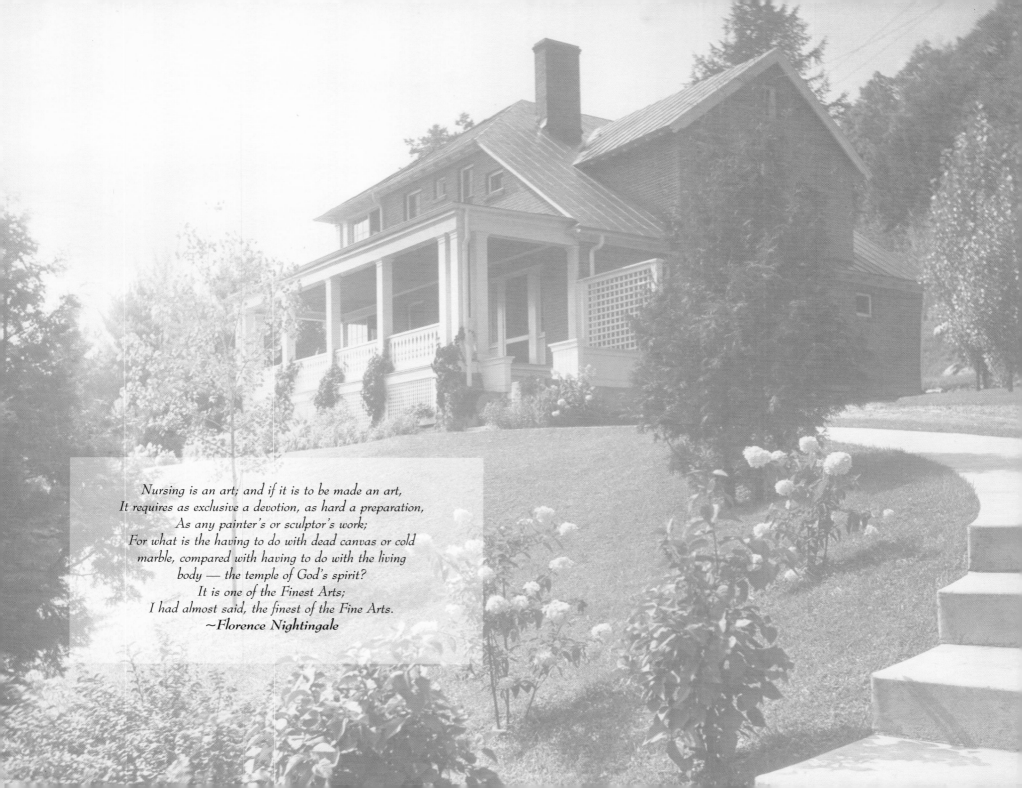

Nursing is an art; and if it is to be made an art,
It requires as exclusive a devotion, as hard a preparation,
As any painter's or sculptor's work;
For what is the having to do with dead canvas or cold
marble, compared with having to do with the living
body — the temple of God's spirit?
It is one of the Finest Arts;
I had almost said, the finest of the Fine Arts.
~Florence Nightingale

In Sickness and in Health:
Portrait of a Nurse

*A*lthough the doctors held daily office hours, it was the nurses who were with the most acute patients twenty-four hours a day. It was the nurses who often sat with their patients around the clock in subzero temperatures out on the cure porches.

It was the nurses who offered support and care when patients had to have a lung collapsed or part of the chest wall removed. It was the nurses who held the hands and wiped the tears of patients when loved ones died in the war; or when hearts broke remembering small children left behind at home; or when newly formed friendships between patients ended in death.

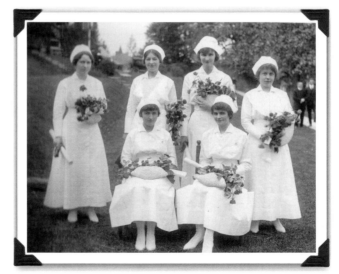

Graduating class of the D. Ogden Mills Training School in 1917
Courtesy of the Trudeau Institute Archives

The nurses were often the same age as their patients. Furthermore, many of the nurses cared for their patients for many months, or even years, before they either got better or died. The majority of practicing nurses at the sanatorium were, themselves, in the process of recovering from TB. Who better to care for someone with TB than one who had been there? All of these factors resulted in a bond between the nurse and the patient that few can imagine or even accurately describe.

Despite the integral role that nurses played in the care of tuberculosis patients, very little has been written about the nursing side of Trudeau Sanatorium. The histories of the nurses who cured and nursed at the sanatorium are wonderfully interesting and, oftentimes, touching. Sadly, much of that historical information was never recorded or, if recorded, has been lost. Fortunately, however, there are a few nurses who are still vital, healthy, and willing to augment the paucity of archival information with personal recollections of their years at the sanatorium. However, in order to provide a backdrop for those stories, an overview will be provided of what nursing was like around the time that the Adirondack Cottage Sanitarium accepted its first two patients in 1884.

Overview of Nursing During the Second Half of the Nineteenth Century

Until the 1860s, the women who provided nursing care were considered to be among the lowest echelon of society. They were:

> *illiterate, rough, and inconsiderate, oftentimes immoral or alcoholic. When a woman could no longer earn a living from gambling or vice, she might become a nurse. Nurses were often drawn from among discharged patients, prisoners, and the lowest strata of society.* [1]

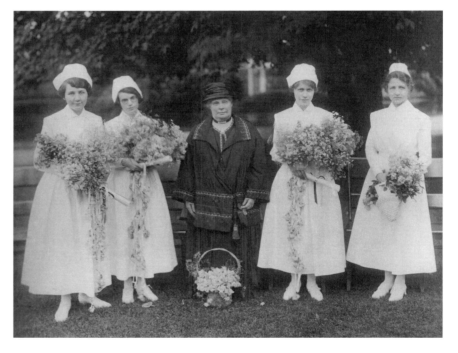

Graduating class of the D. Ogden Mills Training School with Mrs. Whitelaw Reid in 1924
Courtesy of the Trudeau Institute Archives

The Civil War, however, gave an immense boost to nursing. Prior to 1860, there were basically no trained nurses in America. Volunteers, who were self-taught, gave any nursing care that was provided. During the war, hospitals offered quick and intensive courses to any women that would take them, and the religious orders opened their wards to war workers. It became patently evident that the volunteer system of nursing was, at best, inadequate. This paved the way for much needed reform. In 1869 a report was issued to the American Medical Association by one of its subcommittees on the Training of Nurses. The report declared that nursing was as much an exact science as was medicine and urged the establishment, in hospitals, of training schools for nurses. It further suggested that these schools be sponsored and controlled by the medical profession. The report fell on deaf ears.[2]

A few years earlier, Florence Nightingale, on the other side of the ocean, had developed a passion for nursing and social reform. Even as a child, she would nurse her relatives back to health whenever the situation allowed. Her parents, however, refused to allow her to become a nurse as they considered it an unsuitable choice for a woman of her education, wealth, and social position. Finally, in 1851, they relented permitting Florence to journey from England to Germany where she participated in a three-month period of training in nursing at the Deaconess Institute at Kaiserswerth. The full program of study at Kaiserswerth took three years and included:

> A rotation in hospital clinical services (experience on wards for men, women, and children, as well as on wards for communicable disease, convalescents, and sick deaconesses), instruction in visiting nursing, theoretical and bedside instruction in the care of the sick, instruction in religious doctrine and ethics, and enough pharmacy to pass the state examinations for pharmacists. . . . An interesting principle was enforced in that the nurses were required to follow the physician's orders exactly and that the physician alone was responsible for the outcome.[3]

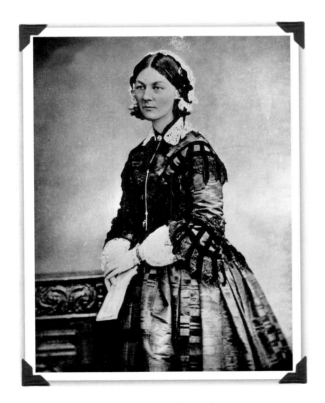

Florence Nightingale
©The Florence Nightingale Museum

Although her training at Kaiserswerth was her only formal nurse's training, Florence later held that the nursing there was crude and that the hospital was the poorest part of the deaconess institution. Therefore, Florence was mostly self-taught, her standards exacting, and her self-expectations nothing short of perfection.

In 1854, during the Crimean War, her friend Sir Sidney Herbert, Britain's Secretary of War, appointed Florence to oversee the introduction of female nurses into the military hospitals in Turkey. Although, at that time, it was unheard of for women who were not in religious orders to involve themselves in army nursing, Florence, with a staff of forty nurses, was able to introduce sanitary science into the military hospitals, thereby reducing the mortality rate from forty-two to two percent. She wrote in a private note, "I stand at the altar of murdered men, and, while I live, I fight their cause."[4]

Out of gratitude for her war efforts, the British government gave Florence enough money so that she could establish the Nightingale Training School at St. Thomas Hospital in London, which opened in 1860. Trained nurses graduating from this school were sent to hospitals in Britain and abroad to establish other training schools based on the Nightingale model.

Also in 1860, Florence published her well-known book, *Notes on Nursing: What It Is and What It Is Not*, which is still in print today and has been translated into at least eleven foreign languages. This little book offers her principles on nursing, which were based on careful observation and extreme sensitivity to the needs of the patients.

Although Trudeau and Nightingale were only a generation apart in age, there is no evidence to suggest that either knew of the other. However, it is interesting to note the many similarities that existed between Florence's beliefs that were recorded in her book and those of Dr. Edward Livingston Trudeau. Most of Dr. Trudeau's initial beliefs regarding healing were based on his "auto-suggestion," observation of his personal experiences in the wilderness, and the scientific experiments that he performed in his little laboratory. Similarly, many of Nightingale's beliefs stemmed from her finely honed intuition, acute powers of observation, and her personal standards and tests.

The following segments taken from her book illustrate the parallel thinking that existed between Nightingale and Trudeau.

On fresh air:

The very first canon of nursing, the first and the last thing upon which a nurse's attention must be fixed, the first essential to a patient, without which all the rest you can do for him is nothing . . . is this: To keep the air he breathes as pure as the external air, without chilling him.

On night air:

Another extraordinary fallacy is the dread of night air. What air can we breathe at night but night air? Fully one-half of all the diseases we suffer from is occasioned by people sleeping with their windows shut. An open window most nights in the year can never hurt any one.

On sunlight:

Therefore, they should be able, to see out of window from their beds, to see sky and sunlight at least, if you can show them nothing else, I assert to be if not the very first importance for recovery, at least something very near it . . . where there is sun, there is thought.

On viewing the outdoors:

They let him lie there staring at a dead wall, without any change of object to enable him to vary his thoughts; and it never even occurs to them, at least to move his bed so that he can look out of the window. . . . In many diseases, especially in convalescence from fever, that wall will appear to make all sorts of faces at him; now flowers never do this.

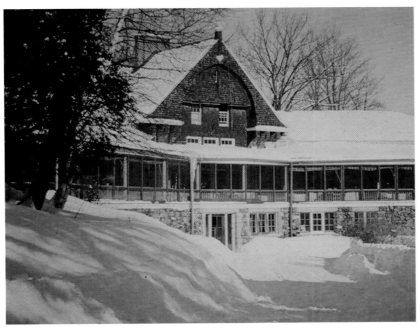

Childs Infirmary showing porches onto which patients' beds were wheeled for their daily treatments of air
Courtesy of the Trudeau Institute Archives

On mind/body effect of environment:

People say the effect is only on the mind. It is no such thing. The effect is on the body, too. Little as we know about the way in which we are affected by form, by colour, by light, we do know this, that they have an actual physical effect.

On supplying some sort of manual labor:

Now you can have no idea of the relief which manual labour is to you. . . . A little needle-work, a little writing, a little cleaning, would be the greatest relief the sick could have.

On cheerfulness:

I incline to think that the majority of cheerful cases is to be found among those patients who are not confined to one room, whatever their suffering, and that the majority of depressed cases will be seen among those subjected to a long monotony of objects about them.

On food:

Milk and the preparation from milk, are a most important article of food for the sick. . . . There is nearly as much nourishment in half a pint of milk as there is in a quarter of a lb. of meat. . . . The diet which will keep the healthy man healthy, will kill the sick one. . . . I should therefore say that incomparably the most important office of the nurse, after she has taken care of the patient's air, is to take care to observe the effect of his food, and report it to the medical attendant.[5]

Meanwhile, back in the United States, the experiences during the Civil War continued to emphasize the critical need to develop organized programs for the training of nurses. Following the largely ignored report to the American Medical Association in 1869, requesting the need for training schools, Mrs. Joseph Hobson, Mrs. William Osborn, and others helped to form the New York State Charities Aid Association and a subcommittee called the Bellevue Hospital Visiting Committee in 1872. This committee inspected the wards at Bellevue Hospital and, finding the conditions deplorable, became a major force behind hospital reform, which included the improvement of nursing. Mrs. Hobson described the conditions that were discovered at Bellevue as follows:

> The "nurses" were prisoners arrested for drunkenness, immorality, or other misdemeanor, who slept in the bathrooms on straw beds laid on the floor, terrorized the helpless sick, took fees, and were not to be trusted with medicines, nor with food brought in by visitors.[6]

This committee ultimately sent Dr. Gill Wylie, a member of the Bellevue medical staff, to Florence Nightingale to elicit her advice and to obtain from her essentials that should be considered when developing a good training school for nurses. The following lists some of those essentials:

> A year's practical and technical training in hospital wards, under trained head nurses who themselves have been trained to train.

> The training of probationers should be as much a part of the duty of the head nurse as directing the under-nurses or seeing to the patients.

> Clinical lectures from the hospital professors . . . elementary instruction in chemistry . . . physiology . . . and general instruction on medical and surgical topics; examinations, written and oral, at least four of each in the year, all adapted to nurses, as also lectures and demonstrations with anatomical, chemical and other illustrations, adapted especially to nurses.

> A good nurses' library of professional books, not for the probationers to skip and dip in at random, but to be made careful use of, under the medical instructor and class-mistress . . . . The authority and discipline over all the women of a trained lady-superintendent . . . who is herself the best nurse in the hospital, the example and leader of her nurses in all that she wishes her nurses to be.

> Accommodations for sleeping, classes, and meals; arrangements for time and teaching and work; surroundings of a moral and religious, and hard-working and sober, yet cheerful tone and atmosphere, such as to make the training-school and hospital a "home" which no good young woman of any class need fear by entering to lose anything of health of body or mind; with moral

and spiritual helps, and an elevating and motherly influence over all, such as to make the whole place which will train really good women, who can withstand temptation and do real work, and neither be "romantic" nor "menial."[7]

Although Wylie did not personally confer with Nightingale while he was in England, he did study her schools. Upon his return to New York, he received a letter from her offering support on the establishment of a school and stressing the point that nurses and physicians have different types of practice and, accordingly, must render different aspects of care. Finally, after overcoming opposition to the establishment of a school and raising the necessary funds, the Bellevue School of Nursing was opened in May of 1873 — the very month and year that young Edward Trudeau made his first journey into the wilderness after being diagnosed with tuberculosis. Although it was at Bellevue where Trudeau's diagnosis of tuberculosis was first made, the strong influence that the Bellevue School of Nursing was later to have on his little world of healing in Saranac Lake was certainly unknown to him at that time.

The Bellevue School of Nursing was the first of three schools based on the Nightingale model that opened in 1873. The Connecticut Training School in New Haven opened its doors in October and the Boston Training School (later called the Massachusetts General Hospital Training School for Nurses) opened in November of that same year. Bellevue, however, became one of the foremost schools in the country and graduated many eminent nursing leaders including Isabel Hampton Robb

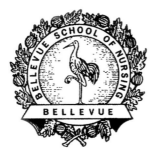

The Bellevue Seal, which was also the school's pin, was designed by Tiffany and Company and adopted in 1880 by the Board of Managers
Courtesy of the Bellevue Alumnae Center for Nursing History, Foundation of The New York State Nurses Association

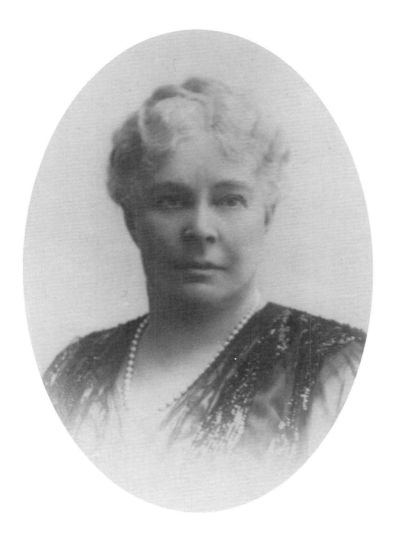

Mrs. Whitelaw Reid
Courtesy of the Trudeau Institute Archives

and Lavinia Lloyd Dock. The schools were obviously a success because by 1879 there were eleven training schools in the country and by 1900 the number had grown to over 400.

Mrs. Whitelaw Reid, who would also play an integral role in the development of nursing at Trudeau's sanatorium in 1912, was one of the early board members of the training school at Bellevue. Her father, D. Ogden Mills, later founded the first male training school in the country called the Mills School for Male Nurses at Bellevue Hospital in 1888. Seemingly random bits of history that were unfolding in New York City would later set into motion a series of events at Trudeau Sanatorium that would become inexorably entwined in the growth, development, and provision of its nursing care.

Before venturing back inside the grounds of Trudeau Sanatorium to take a closer look at the nurses of Trudeau, a few other nursing historical landmarks should be mentioned. Many of the student nurses were sent from the hospital training schools into private homes to care for wealthy patients who could afford to pay the hospitals for private duty nurses. Initially, calls were placed to the hospital when seeking a private nurse. Later, the training schools organized their own nursing registries for that purpose, and finally the nurses themselves centralized the service which gave birth to the concept of visiting nursing, as it was called, in 1877. Miss Effie Benedict, a Bellevue nurse, was the first to establish a non-sectarian nursing service and was considered to be the first American district nurse outside of mission affiliations. In 1886 the first visiting nursing associations were formed in Boston and Philadelphia.

Lillian Wald founded the first known Nurses' Settlement on Henry Street in New York City in 1893. It was Wald's nursing settlement concept that helped to expand the scope of visiting nursing into the larger arena of what she termed "public health nursing." Wald created a system "whereby patients had direct access to nurses and nurses had direct access to patients. Wald insisted that the nurses should be at the call of people who needed them, without the intervention of a medical man."[8] A variation of this form of nursing would later become evident at the Adirondack Cottage Sanitarium.

As one additional point of reference, recall that in 1889 Dr. Hermann Biggs urged New York City to actively campaign against tuberculosis. Four years later, in 1893, Lillian Wald, in one of her major efforts at prevention, was the first to supply sputum cups and disinfectants to pioneer tuberculosis nurses.

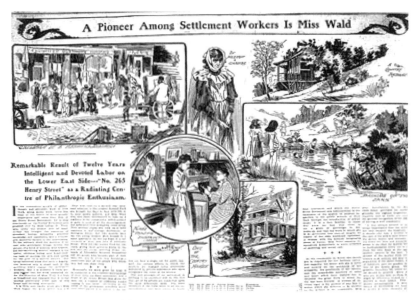

Wald Article on Sunday, April 23, 1905
Courtesy of the New York Times

The Pioneer Nurses of Trudeau

It took a relatively short time for the rapid changes that were occurring in nursing to find their way into the wilderness of Trudeau's pioneer sanatorium that was so quickly developing in Saranac Lake. Up until 1893, when the little infirmary cottage had been built, the only "nurses" Trudeau had available were the guides and lumberman to care for the male patients, and "any old women I could get" to take care of the female patients. Finally, in 1893, he hired Miss Ruth Collins, who became not only the first nurse to work at the sanatorium, but also an extremely giving, much loved, and respected individual.

Ruth Collins was born in England in 1863 and arrived in Saranac Lake in 1893 to become the infirmary nurse at the Adirondack Cottage Sanitarium. Miss Collins remained at the sanatorium until November of 1908 at which time she left to ultimately operate her own nursing cure cottage, the Collins Cottage, on Park Avenue in Saranac Lake. Dr Trudeau had the following words to say at her farewell celebration:

We are gathered here tonight to say an official farewell and express our good wishes, and to honor a tried and trusted comrade who for many years has borne with us the heat and burden of the day in the work of this institution.

I want to express to Miss Collins, for Mrs. Trudeau and myself, for the management, the doctors, and all who have been associated with her here, the deep regret we feel at her leaving the Sanitarium to take up a new work in the village. The early history of the Sanitarium's struggle for existence if it is ever written would show a long record of self-sacrificing devotion by all those who labored here with me so many years for its establishment. Miss Collins has done her full share to this end and to make the Sanitarium what it is today, not only in the opportunities it offers for restoration to health, but in the spirit of its work as well.

Miss Collins began her work here in an old infirmary where she was the only nurse, and for years, no matter how crowded it might be, she did all the work, being on duty both night and day, and those who have been in her care know full well that she never spares herself, and how tender and skillful are her ministrations. She has been with us now for fifteen years! How many of us can lay claim in a life time to as much hard work done for others and as many good deeds as she has crowded into those fifteen years? She has taught me many lessons in the great gospel of unselfishness, and I will never forget her coming to me a long while ago to ask if she might, as a favor, be allowed to bring from the village a hopeless case, a man in the last stages of consumption who was both friendless and penniless, in order that she might nurse him until the end. This she did, putting him in her own room and sleeping for three months herself on the lounge in the sitting room, doing

Handwritten text of Dr. Trudeau's farewell speech to Ruth Collins in 1908
Courtesy of the Adirondack Collection, Saranac Free Library

meanwhile all her usual work as well. Now ladies and gentlemen, few of us ever get as far as this, and I confess that ever since I have had a most chastened opinion of my own attempts in the same direction.

We admire Miss Collins for her good work and her good deeds. We love her for herself, and we want her to know it. We are very glad she is not going to leave Saranac Lake and will not pass entirely out of our lives. We bid her farewell with very full hearts, and God-speed in the new work she is entering upon.[9]

While Trudeau's sanatorium was undergoing continuous expansion on the inside, Saranac Lake was becoming rapidly transformed on the outside. Numerous entrepreneurs, many of whom were nurses, opened houses or cottages in the village as private sanatoria, most with capacities of fewer than twenty patients. In a relatively short time, the entire village was transformed into a cottage industry. Although not all the cure cottages were run by nurses, the nursing cottages provided the most intensive care of the cottages and were considered to be more demanding, requiring more resources, expertise, and equipment than were the boarding cottages. After leaving the sanatorium, Ruth Collins purchased and operated a cross-gabled Queen Anne house at 76 Park Avenue in Saranac Lake. It had a capacity of ten and became known as the Collins Cottage.[10]

A second nurse began her practice at the sanatorium in 1899. Three months before Mary Burgess was to finish her nurse's training in Michigan, she was discovered to have an incipient lesion on her lung. Although she tried to convince the doctor that he was wrong, she failed, and soon entered the Adirondack Cottage Sanitarium. She was to become the first cottage nurse, which was not unlike the public health nursing concept developed by Lillian Wald six years earlier. As a cottage nurse, she would visit the patients on the grounds to perform any required nursing treatments and assessments, offer counseling services and prevention strategies, as well as teach disease management. This was the first

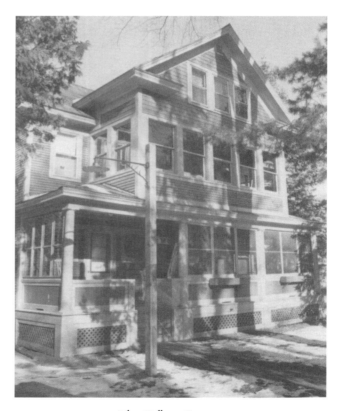

The Collins Cottage
Courtesy of Philip L. Gallos and Historic Saranac Lake

time that the patients, living on the grounds had access to the professional services of a nurse. Most of the nursing provided was based on the nurses' personal experiences with TB, on the care they received while patients at the sanatorium, and on the teachings of Drs. Trudeau and Brown. What follows is Mary's fond recollection of the time she spent at the sanatorium.

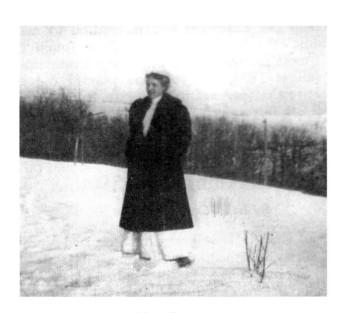

Mary Burgess
"Journal of the Outdoor Life"

To meet with Dr. Trudeau was to be inspired with confidence in him, and to become acquainted with and to work with him I have counted one of my blessings. He was beloved by all, patients and non-patients alike. I arrived in Saranac Lake in October 1899, much depressed, but was made to feel at home almost immediately. On the contrary, I very shortly realized my illness was to be a blessing in disguise.

I went to Saranac Lake fully expecting to return to Michigan to resume my nursing work after three months. But for eighteen months I did practically nothing but take the cure. Under the excellent medical direction of Dr. Trudeau and his assistants, and the untiring care of Miss Ruth Collins, at that time the only nurse in the Sanitorium, I finally was able to take up my work by first assisting Miss Collins in the infirmary. Later Dr. Lawrason Brown conceived the idea that it would be an advantage to have a nurse to visit and care for patients who lived in the cottages but who were slightly indisposed, and I was asked to take up this work. I was glad to do this, and thus started the cottage nursing at Trudeau.

*Among the patients, at least during my residence, there was a wonderful spirit of good cheer, which would do anybody's heart good. This combined with the careful supervision of all in authority, and as a background the bracing air of the pine-scented Adirondacks, the scenery and the sunsets — well! Patients **just must get well** at Trudeau.*[11]

In 1900 it was through the efforts of a local clergyman that a trained nurse was secured for the purpose of answering emergency calls and performing district nursing at the request of physicians in town requiring her assistance. This marked the beginning of the Saranac Lake District Nursing Association.

Agnes Kernan, a cottage nurse at the sanatorium in 1902, tells of some of her experiences at Trudeau. Agnes received her training at Johns Hopkins training school, which was opened in 1889 under Isabel Hampton Robb. Again, her experience mirrors the public health nursing concept of Wald, as she clearly details the direct contact she had with her patients as well as the many nursing interventions that were allowed her without a doctor's order.

> The cottage nurse has charge of the cottage patients, makes rounds, attends to the sick in the cottages and tents, sends meals to those unable to come to the dining room and is sent for if anything happens. . . . The variety of treatment is limited, for it must be remembered that only incipient cases are supposed to be admitted; however statistics for 1902 show that of 142 patients admitted, only 28 percent were incipient, 69 percent advanced and 1 percent doubtful cases. Pleurisy, colds, hemorrhages and high temperatures are the usual troubles found and the ways of meeting these are few. Rubbing with liniments, painting with iodine, strapping or simple applications may be used for pleurisy without the doctor's order. In hemorrhage ice internally and to the heart, small doses of morphia or codeia hypodermically if necessary, may be given before the doctor arrives. Occasionally other emergencies are to be met. Once when answering a call, and going preparing for a hemorrhage, I found a patient suffering from a gunshot wound through the foot! Cut fingers, badly burned fingers from upset candy stews, and similar accidents prevent one's forgetting the technique of a surgical dressing.

> The rules are few and pertain so closely to the patient's welfare, they are usually kept without requiring to be enforced. During the first week of residence, the patient's temperature is taken and recorded morning and night, and afterwards when elevated. Those having an evening temperature of 99.5 degrees are kept in bed until it has been normal at least two days. The diet consists largely of meat, eggs and milk with vegetables and sweetmeats to tempt the appetite. Those unable to eat the general diet are provided with extra quantities of milk and eggs and each patient is given a half pint of milk before retiring. The patients are weighed every two weeks and weight

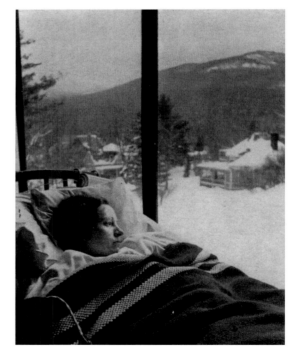

Taking the air on a cottage veranda
Alfred Eisenstadt/TimePix

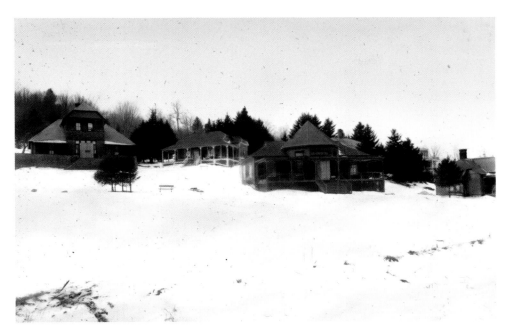

charts are kept. The gain is usually rapid and sometimes as much as five or six pounds in a week. . . . All are required to spend eight to ten hours a day in the open air; many sleep on the verandas even in severe weather and some live in tents from May until November.

Those who expectorate are provided with sputum cups, a box made of heaviest paper, having the edges so folded inward as to make a funnel-shaped opening through which to expectorate and thus lessoning the danger of the sputum being spilt. The boxes are fitted in covered brass frames. Patients are taught how to carbolize the frames and when it becomes necessary to change the box, it is wrapped securely in paper, placed in covered receptacles which are collected daily. Expectorating in handkerchiefs and cloths is strictly prohibited.

The cottage system has its disadvantages, we grant. It is impossible to watch the patient as in hospital wards . . . but this plan obviates the evils of many persons in one building, and from the patient's view, is certainly to be preferred. A patient once said to me she had had the comforts of a home without its responsibility. As to danger of infection, it is reduced to a minimum. No case has ever developed in the Sanitarium, and many of the employees have worked for years in the dining-room and cottages without ill effects.

These facts are evident — the treatment prolongs life, teaches the unfortunate how to live, and how to protect himself and the non-infected by proper care and disposal of infectious materials; and only when the people realize and practice these laws can the great white plague be mastered.[12]

Madeline Smith, who was a graduate of St. Luke's Hospital in Chicago, described some of the changes that had occurred at the sanatorium by 1909 when she was part of the nursing staff:

If any nurse thinks of contracting tuberculosis, may a kind Providence send her to the Adirondack Cottage Sanitarium.

The staff at Trudeau consists of the physician in charge, a lady superintendent, two assistant physicians, a head nurse, and three assistant nurses. The head nurse, with one assistant, is in charge of the infirmary, while the remaining two attend to the cottage nursing. This number of nurses is sufficient to meet all ordinary demands of the hundred or more patients.

It is a noteworthy fact that all the positions at the sanitarium are filled by former patients or those who at one time or another have had tuberculosis.

The statistics of the Adirondack Cottage Sanitarium show most satisfying results of the treatment in vogue there. The gratitude of hundreds of people is due to the tireless efforts of Dr. Trudeau and the friends who have helped him in his work. . . . Numerous other institutions for the same cause have [now] been established, none however with a more beautiful setting or showing a better record of health. It has made the names of Trudeau and Saranac Lake famous the world over. [13]

D. Ogden Mills Training School for Nurses

It was becoming increasing difficult to hire hospital-trained nurses who would be willing to take care of the tuberculosis patients at the sanatorium. Some hospitals were even said to use assignment of nurses to the TB wards as a form of punishment.

The rapid increase in the number of special institutions for the tuberculous has coincided with a steady decrease in the supply of nurses available and willing to care for such patients. No inducements are made for the highly trained nurses to enter this field. It offers little attraction to the more ambitious young women who like action and variety. Nursing the chronic tuberculosis patient excited no enthusiasm in them. In fact, few have had any training in or contact with tuberculosis except in its terminal stages, and these few only when serving in some large general hospital having special departments for chronic cases. Such contact fails utterly to inspire the pupil nurse; rather it fills her with dread. [14]

It was evident that some other provision had to be made if the sanatorium was to provide the level of care consistent with the needs of the ever-growing patient population. As successful training schools had been in existence at other sanatoria for several years, in 1912 Dr. Trudeau decided that the time had come to establish such a school at his sanatorium. It was felt that the young women at the sanatorium whose disease had been arrested would be perfect candidates for the training school.

The arrested case of tuberculosis is peculiarly well fitted to nursing the tuberculosis patient, not only because of her personal experience with the disease which develops sympathy with and appreciation of the patient's mental attitude, but also because the mere fact that she has had and has overcome the disease supplies an object lesson to the patient and gives encouragement and hope to an individual who is in constant need of such an example through the long, tedious, and oftentimes discouraging period of recovery.

It has been said that the monotony of tuberculosis nursing tends to make the worker "stale" after two or three years. This is not true of the specially trained tuberculosis nurse. Her interest and enthusiasm grow with the years. There is no foundation for the fear that she will migrate into the field of general nursing. In her own field she is finding so much and such interesting work and she realizes only too well that "the harvest indeed is great but the laborers are few." The demands at all times for such workers far exceed the supply.

If at the end of her career a tuberculosis nurse can say she has succeeded in impressing upon twenty-five careless people the necessity of preventive measures, she not only feels that she has helped to overcome the tuberculosis bacillus, but has also helped to diminish the mortality of the next generation. [15]

By the turn of the century, training schools were becoming almost crucial to the running of a hospital. The presence of nursing students improved the quality of care that was given to patients and also had a positive impact on the cost of the provision of that care. In fact, many hospitals established schools of nursing for the sole purpose of using the students to provide cost effective care to its patients. The students worked long tedious hours in payment for the schooling that they were receiving at the hospital.

At Trudeau Sanatorium, unlike many of the metropolitan hospitals, the motives for starting a little training school for nurses were solely altruistic. Although it is true that many of the nurses graduating from the school did stay on to provide nursing care for the sanatorium, that was far from Dr. Trudeau's primary objective. He believed that for those individuals that demonstrated a natural ability for nursing as a career, his school would firstly serve as an important component of occupational therapy by providing the students an important means of following a useful life, and, secondly, by educating the students in the modern treatment of tuberculosis, provide a service that was so severely lacking in the rest of the country. The graduates from his nursing program were in demand throughout the country. Some of the students had already started a nursing program elsewhere, and upon contracting TB, came to the sanatorium where they could regain their health and earn a living as a TB nurse at the same time. Others came for the cure, and once they were in an arrested state, decided to stay on and enroll in the little training school.

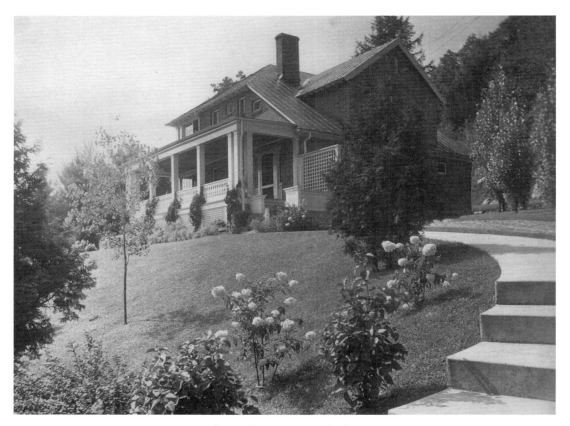

D. Ogden Mills Training School in 1912
Courtesy of the Trudeau Institute Archives

Looking backward through the lens of time, it is interesting to observe how seemingly effortlessly so many of Dr. Trudeau's innovative ideas were turned into reality. It was as though Dr. Trudeau, without knowing it, engendered in others his contagion of giving. In this case the large heart with equally large hands belonged to Mrs. Whitelaw Reid who knew Dr. Trudeau through her frequent summering at St. Regis. She was the daughter of Darius Ogden Mills, a "forty-niner" who helped to form the Bank of California. Her husband, Whitelaw Reid, was the editor of the *New York Tribune* and ambassador of the United States at the Court of St. James having been so appointed by Theodore Roosevelt.

Mrs. Reid was internationally known in her own right for her magnanimous philanthropy. She built the San Mateo Hospital near San Francisco as a memorial to her parents "equipping it with the latest in scientific apparatus and enveloping it in an atmosphere of cheerfulness." She also, with her brother, was instrumental in building St. Luke's Hospital in San Francisco; and helped to form the London Chapter of the American Red Cross. In 1922 the French government conferred upon her the Cross of Chevalier of the Legion of Honor in recognition of her many benefactions to the people of France.[16]

In 1911 Mrs. Whitelaw Reid donated $10,000 for the purchase of a nurse's cottage at Trudeau's sanatorium that was to be named the D. Ogden Mills Training School, in memory of her father.

In this substantial and comfortable little brick structure each [of six nurses] has her own bedroom, her own dressing closet with

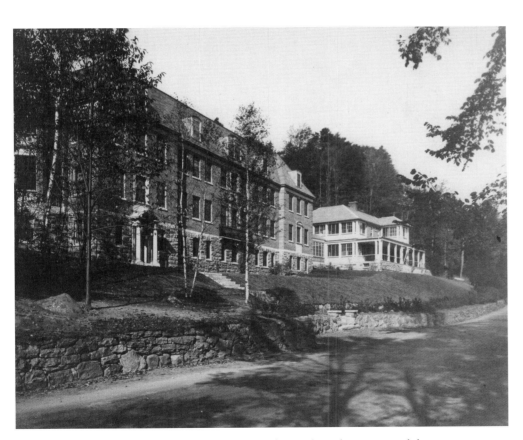

D. Ogden Mills Training School (on right) and Reid House (on left) in 1930
Courtesy of the Trudeau Institute Archives

running water, and a sleeping porch with a southern exposure where she can carry out the open air treatment which is still essential for most of the pupil nurses. On the lower floor is a homelike sitting room with a large open fireplace where the nurses can meet when off duty.[17]

Mrs. Reid donated an additional $150,000 in 1930, for the purpose of remodeling the training school and constructing Reid House, which was regarded as the most modern and fully equipped home for nurses in the United States. The new building contained:

rooms for twenty-three pupil nurses and suites of rooms with bath for six head nurses and one supervisor, as well as one guest room and two maids' rooms. Public rooms include a lecture hall, diet kitchen, demonstration diet kitchen, large living room, reception room and library.[18]

The D. Ogden Mills Training School accepted its first three pupils in 1912, under the direction of Miss Wadland, the superintendent of nurses. At that time, in order to be accepted, the students had to have had TB and be in an arrested state prior to admission.

The images on pages 126-134 were taken from various annual reports and class notes that were all contained in the *Scrapbook on the D. Ogden Mills School of Nursing* located in the Trudeau Institute Archives.

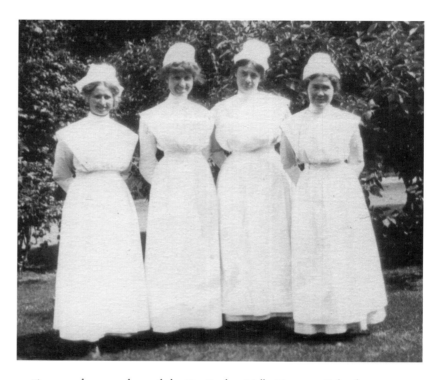

First graduating class of the D. Ogden Mills Training School in 1914. From left to right: Miss Colgate; Miss Wadland, Superintendent; Miss Van Heckle; and Miss Kane.
Courtesy of the Trudeau Institute Archives

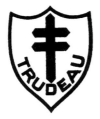

When the first three young women to train at Trudeau desired a pin and school seal, they chose one similar to that of the first superintendent of nurses — a Maltese cross on a blunt shield. Our predecessors in training chose for this school the Florentine cross in garnet red, and fitted it to a narrower shield of white. Only a decade before, this cross had been used for the first time to symbolise interest in tuberculosis control.

It is singular to note that the very year (1912) which saw its adoption by this training school, also saw the first definite move to confine its use to accredited tuberculosis work and interests, and the Florentine cross with its double bar became the recognised standard for all those engaged in the fight to control and eradicate the white plague.

Our school motto, "Comfort Often, Relieve Always" appears on the back of our pins, and is carved on the memorial to Dr. Trudeau, whose personal motto it was. As nurses we do well to leave the aggressive fight against the causes and source of disease to the doctors and scientists, and ourselves carry on the daily command to

"COMFORT OFTEN; RELIEVE ALWAYS"

1929 D. Ogden Mills School of Nursing Handbook

Notes from Dr. Trudeau's 1913 Annual Report read:

The nurses training school has been in operation during the past year. Most of the time under the superintendence of Edith Wadland [later replaced by Miss Roberts]. On October 1, the first 3 specially trained tuberculosis nurses were graduated with appropriate exercises at the sanitarium. These young women all had had their diseases arrested while patients in the institution and had remained well throughout the 2 years necessary for them to obtain their degree. Two of them at once secured positions, the third is still working at the sanatorium. Thus the sanatorium not only restored their health but has trained them to an independent career of usefulness. The school now has 8 pupil nurses under training.

The specially trained tuberculosis nurse is well fitted for a work which the regular trained nurse generally refuses to undertake. She is familiar with all the details of treatment generally employed for the relief of the patient's symptoms. She is able to act promptly and intelligently in case of emergency and in the absence of the physician. She is fitted to educate the invalid and his family as to where the danger of infection lies and how to avert it. We have certainly progressed in the nursing of tuberculosis at the sanatorium. For I can look back on the early days at the institution when the patients had to be nursed by old women from the village, guides, and lumberman, as I could get them.[19]

Requirements for Entrance

Education

Under the laws of New York State, a student must have at least one year High School work, or its equivalent.

Age

Applicant should be between the ages of eighteen and thirty-five years.

Health

A satisfactory report of your general physical condition by your own physician, and a chest examination by one of our examining physicians. (Name of the nearest examining physician will be sent on request).

Application

Application blanks will be sent on request, when a personal interview cannot be arranged. A recent photograph should be returned with application.

General Information

Illness

In illness all pupils are cared for gratuitously for two months, but all time lost in excess of two weeks a year must be made up.

Remuneration

An allowance of $10 a month after acceptance into the school.

Equipment

When accepted into the school, students are allowed three uniforms, eight aprons, twelve bibs, two caps, and the loan of students' books. Complete directions for making probationary uniforms, aprons, etc., are sent when student is accepted.

Maintenance

Room and board are provided.

Laundry

A reasonable amount of laundry is done free.

1923-1924 Entry Requirements and General Information

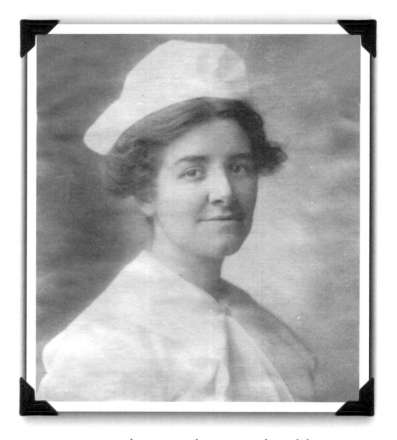

Miss Roberts, second Superintendent of the D. Ogden Mills Training School, in 1913

Course of training covers two years and in addition the pupils in satisfactory health may affiliate with a general hospital of good standing. A schedule of course follows:

Theory

First Year

FIRST SEMESTER — January to April

Preliminary Course, 4 Months	Lectures
Pathology, Anatomy and Physiology	60
Chemistry	16
Bacteriology	16
Hygiene	8
Nutrition and Cookery	36
Hospital Housekeeping	8
Drugs and Solutions	16
Materia Medica	16
Elementary Nursing	54
Bandaging	10
History of Nursing and its Ethical and Social Basis	6
History of Nursing, with Slides	2
	248

SECOND SEMESTER — 2 Months — April to June

Tuberculosis	16
Advanced Nursing (incl. Massage)	32
Diet and Disease	8
Ethics	8
Pyschology	8
Occupational Therapy	8
	80

June to September, No Classes

Second Year or Junior Year

September 4th to June 15th

Internal Medicine, Incl. Eye, Ear, Nose and Throat, Nervous and Mental and Skin and Venereal Diseases	40
Surgery, Gynecology and Obstetrics	32
Occupational Therapy	8
X-ray	32
	112

1923-1924 required nursing courses at the D. Ogden Mills Training School

In keeping with Trudeau and Nightingale's emphasis on the holistic approach to patient care, the courses emphasized cooking, psychology, massage, and occupational therapy. Also recall that Susan Tracy implemented the first occupational nursing program for nurses in 1906. Only six years later, the concept was introduced into the new training school at Trudeau's sanatorium. Once again Trudeau and his pioneer world of healing were on the cutting edge of innovation.

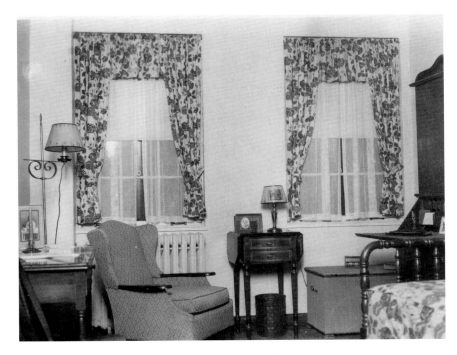

Student nurse's bedroom at Reid House in 1930

It is not known how much influence Mrs. Whitelaw Reid had in the initial organization of the training school. However, as this school was obviously based on the Nightingale model, it would be a fair assumption to conclude that Mrs. Reid, who had significant experience as a board member of the Bellevue School of Nursing, left her fingerprint on the early development of the school. In reviewing the course descriptions, as well as the pictures of the home-like environment that was provided the student nurses, there is no doubt that Miss Nightingale would have approved. Every one of the Nightingale essentials previously described had been included in this little training school.

The Florence Nightingale Pledge

I solemnly pledge myself before God and in the presence of this assembly to pass my life in purity and to practice my profession faithfully. I will abstain from whatever is deleterious and mischievous, and will not take or knowingly administer any harmful drug. I will do all in my power to elevate the standard of my profession, and will hold in confidence all personal matters committed to my keeping, and all family affairs coming to my knowledge in the practice of my calling. With loyalty will I endeavor to aid the physician in his work and devote myself to the welfare of those committed to my care.

Class of 1929 Handbook

The D. Ogden Mills Training School was registered by the New York State Board of Regents in 1921. This meant "that from then on all applicants to the Training School had to submit records of their preliminary education to The State Department for approval before they could be admitted. It means also that the School is inspected annually by a representative of The Department."[20]

By 1923 students who completed the two-year course and passed all examinations satisfactorily were given a diploma of the school and presented with a Trudeau School pin. They were not allowed to take the State Board Examinations until they had spent an additional year affiliating with a general hospital. Over the years, the students affiliated with the following hospitals: Bellevue Hospital, New York Hospital, Long Island College Hospital, Samaritan Hospital, Yale University School of Nursing, Manhattan Maternity Hospital, Syracuse Memorial Hospital, and Fordham Hospital.

Graduation day at the G. Ogden Mills Training School was a special time of celebration and tradition. Sophia Palmer, who was editor of *The American Journal of Nursing* from its inception until 1920; and Effie Taylor, who was president of the International Council of Nurses, promoted university based nursing education, and served as the second dean of the Yale School of Nursing; were two of many notables who delivered commencement addresses at the school.

Dr. Beattie Brown gave one of the more moving commencement addresses in 1921:

> *Other and higher motives you might have but one of your motives surely is that you may achieve success in the noble work to which you have chosen to devote yourselves. At the onset let me suggest that you banish from your mind the idea that success consists in doing something of a very exceptional or spectacular nature that may secure a temporary reputation. But remember what goes up like a rocket comes down like a stick. Reputation is like the crest on the wave — the next instant it is gone. Like the uncertainty of wind that drives the sailing vessel — only a squall and it's dead. Reputation is like the meteor lights that march across the sky and then sink in the deep dark of night. While success is like the steady morning star that shines on and on until it is absorbed and lost in the brightness and glory of the coming day. Success is the favorable accomplishment of what one attempts to do and is only satisfying*

to its possessor as it is made for the instrument for helping others and herein lies the nobleness of your profession. There are occasions that come to all of us when we see sights that we think are grand. I have seen at midnight the headlight of a giant locomotive rushing onward to the darkness, heedless of danger and uncertainty, and have thought the sight grand. I have seen the light come over an eastern hill in glory driving the lazy darkness like mist before a sea born gale til leaf and tree and blade of grass sparkled in the myriad diamonds of the morning's rays. And I have thought it was grand. But at this moment I have in view a

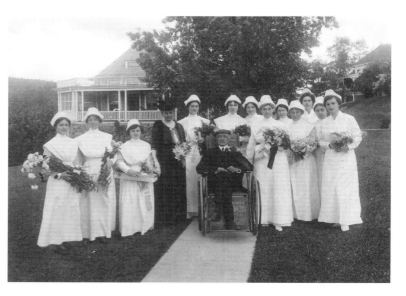

Every year until his death, Dr. and Mrs. Trudeau would have their picture taken with the the graduating class. This picture was taken with the 1915 graduating class the year of his death. After his death, Mrs. Trudeau continued to be present for the annual class photograph.

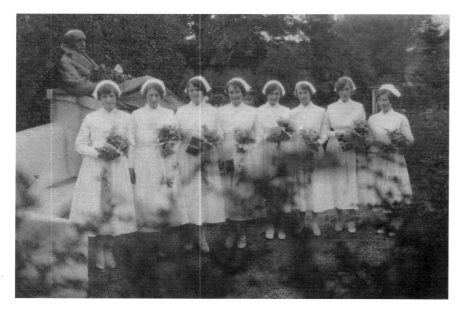

Each year, since the unveiling of the statue commemorating Dr. Trudeau in 1918, immediately following the graduation exercises, the nurses would go to the Trudeau monument for the annual ceremony of placing flowers in Dr. Trudeau's lap as their memorial to the founder of their school.

sight grander than them all. Grander because it is a crisis of life. The vision of you members of the graduating class rising as it were like the lights from among those hills of Trudeau sending the rays of your influence far out into the deep darkness that enshrouds so many of our human kind. And by the tender touch of those rays, of your thought, your devotion, your care, your skill, dispelling that darkness and in its place letting in the light of a new hope, a brighter day to those whose hope had vanished in the gloom.[21]

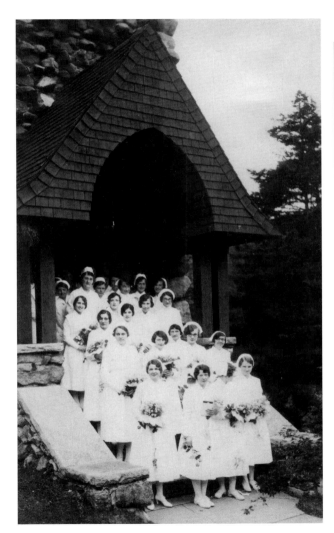

Class of 1929 at Baker Chapel

Class History.

Two years have passed and now we have come to the end of our nursing course. In retrospect, these years seem brief but how different it appeared when we began the grind under the guidance of Miss Amberson. The first month was to most of us a bewildering nightmare. There was always that fear which comes after the immediate arrest of tuberculosis that we would break again. Great was our rejoicing when after a few brief months we began to see that we were able to work again and that we could also keep up our studies. Though we were glad to know these facts, lectures and quizzes were not entirely to our liking. We often thought, after working all day in the infirmaries, that study was a bore. However, at the end of our course, we were all glad that we had done well and appreciated the fact that we had absorbed not only knowledge but had learned many lessons of life.

We started our probationary period on August 15, 1927. Will any of us forget with what mingled feelings of pride and chagrin we donned those unbecoming uniforms and crept shyly into our first class. Later we entered the dining room amidst great applause which made us feel that we might be appreciated after all. This was quickly forgotten, however, and our struggle with Anatomy, Hospital Housekeeping, Bacteriology, Practical Nursing, etc. started.

Anatomy was an enigma to most but we forgot all this under the influence of that highly cultured and sympathetic gentleman, Dr. Gardner. Bacteriology was interesting but we found it most disconcerting to learn so much about those little germs called "Bacilli". Hospital Housekeeping would have been unbearable but for our teacher, Miss Sawtell.

In spite of the hard examinations, we all "skinned through". On December 15th we were capped and I wonder how many of us felt as Betty did when with her cap in her hand, she said, "What shall I do with it?"

As we had weathered the storm of the probationary period, we felt distinctly safe till the examinations of Materia Medica, Advanced Nursing, Pathology, etc. approached. Who could forget Dr. Jahn's little sayings and his well-groomed figure as he directed each nurse in turn to the board with that air of — "Do you know your lesson, little girl?"

Then classes ceased and vacation time came and each in turn departed for a rest after an arduous year.

This last year was ushered in with much rejoicing that the worst was over. Two members of the class departed, but we gained two others. The merry whirl of this year was never taken too seriously. Lectures were judged with the utmost candor. The ribald spirit grew more and more pronounced and the class became rather a club with entertainment before lectures never wanting. One class after another flitted past while the steady drone of lectures and work dulled our energies. However, a fertile topic for conversation was always found from our experiences in the wards.

It was during this year that Miss Amberson resigned and was succeeded by Miss Sawtell and she, in turn, was succeeded by Miss Tibbetts as Assistant Superintendent. Under their kind and never-ceasing care, we have gained much. The influence of their personalities will always remain with us and guide us on to better things after we have left these portals which have led us back to health and happiness.

Class of 1929 history

By 1935, one year before the school closed, the following information was available about the alumni:

Total number of graduates of the 2 year course	157
Registered	87
Completing 3rd year	17
Unable or unwilling to affiliate	53
Single	103
Married	41
Dead	13
Doing TB work	62
In Public Health Field	9
General Hospital Work	18

7 are Superintendents of Nurses in Sanatoria
3 are Instructors in General Hospitals
2 are on the teaching staff of the Yale School of Nursing

Alumni Demographics

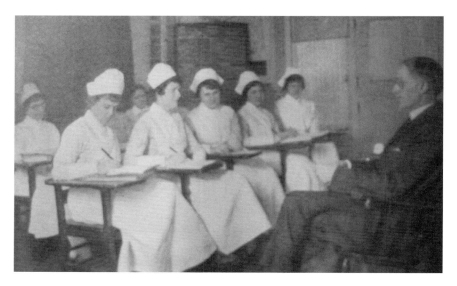

Dr. Baldwin teaching the student nurses

The last class graduated in 1936 and, beginning in the summer of that same year, the sanatorium offered postgraduate courses in tuberculosis nursing for nurses from affiliating hospitals.

> *Because of these changes there will be a larger staff for graduate nurses on general duty than heretofore. The salary is $67.00 per month. Nurses will occupy single rooms at Reid House or Mills Cottage.*[22]

Shortly after the implementation of this noncollegiate clinical program, the following announcement was made:

Word has just been received by Trudeau Sanatorium that the basic noncollegiate program in tuberculosis nursing offered by the Department of Nursing has been approved by the national nursing accrediting service. Trudeau Sanatorium has thus become one of the first sanatoria in the country to have its nursing teaching program receive approval by this national approving body. The course has already been approved by the State Education Department of the University of the State of New York. At the present time 15 students are affiliating at Trudeau from Highland Hospital in Rochester and from Buffalo General Hospital. The course covers a period of 8 weeks and in addition to the basic course at Trudeau includes a 1 week's experienced in thoracic surgery at Saranac General Hospital and clinical experience with the Public Health nurses at Raybrook Sanatorium.[23]

Caring in Ways Remembered: The Nurses' Stories

At eighty years of age, Elizabeth Ann Bell decided it was time to tell her story of nursing and her years at Trudeau Sanatorium. She came to Saranac Lake in 1924, following a bronchial cold from which she was unable to recover. After an examination by Dr. Francis Trudeau, it was decided that Elizabeth had an arrested case of tuberculosis and was given a room in Mrs. Little's cottage, as the sanatorium had no vacancy at the time. Mrs. Little was not a nurse, but "watched over us like a mother hen with baby chickens." Mrs. Little soon took Elizabeth on as her apprentice, teaching her how to record the temperatures on the graphic charts and provide basic care to some of the residents who were on bed rest. A few months later, following a back injury, Mrs. Little asked Elizabeth to take over the care of the patients for a salary of seventy-five dollars a month. After receiving permission from Dr. Trudeau, she agreed to provide the "nursing care" to the residents of Little Cottage.

We admitted patients from time to time, and I became particularly fond of Katherine Bruce, a beautiful nineteen-year-old who was very sick. She had been a sophomore at college and during the Christmas holidays her parents, teenage brother and she stayed in a hotel in New York for a week, where her father had tickets to theaters every night. She gave out and they called a doctor who made the diagnosis, and her mother brought her to Saranac Lake and to us. She was a complete bed patient, so I grew to know her very well. Dr. Trudeau gave her pneumothorax at once, and she responded nicely. Her temperature dropped from 103 to normal, she gained weight, lost her cough, and soon became her delightful self. I think caring for her brought back my desire to become a graduate nurse. Most of our patients recovered to return to their homes and work, but not all, and Katherine's story ended tragically. She had been engaged to a Lee boy in Virginia and had spent days the previous summer on the family yacht on the Potomac. When his family learned of her illness, they insisted that he break the engagement and they took him to Europe the following summer so he wouldn't be tempted to try to see her. That fall she returned to her home in New Jersey, still taking pneumothorax, with instructions to limit her activities. She began to have dates and, in her effort to hide her hurt, overdid and some time later returned to the Little Cottage. She was very sick and this time had disease in both lungs. . . . She died on Christmas Eve.[24]

During the summer of 1926, Elizabeth left Little Cottage and went to work for Dr. Francis Trudeau taking care of his six-year-old son, Frank, who had developed osteomyelitis of the femur. "Mrs. Little was upset, but you didn't say 'No' to the Trudeaus, so I went." She decided to stay with the Trudeaus until the following January when she would enter nursing school at the D. Ogden Mills Training School at the sanatorium.

I lived in Dr. Trudeau's office building in town [which had been Dr. E. L. Trudeau's home and office] where his office nurse lived; and either the Trudeaus or a taxi took me out to their house every morning before breakfast, returning me after dinner in the evening. I assisted Dr. Soper with the dressings and tried to keep Frank entertained and happy. . . . I will never forget that Christmas. When we came down to breakfast the living room doors were closed, and after eating we had to return upstairs until we were called. When we entered the living room, a live pony was tied to the mantelpiece! And I had never seen so many gifts. It seemed that most of Dr. Trudeau's patients sent gifts to the boys. When they were finished opening them, there was a pile of paper higher than I! One gift Frank received was a toy car in pieces with directions for putting it together. They were very clear and I followed them carefully with the result that the car went forward or in reverse by using a gearshift. Dr. Trudeau never got over the fact that a woman could put a car together that would run.[25]

In January of 1926, Elizabeth entered the training school.

We put on our uniforms, aprons, cuffs, and stiff collars and reported for inspection that afternoon. There were eight of us, all of whom had inactive tuberculosis, and one was dropped at once because of health. . . . After one day we were assigned to a floor, and were on duty 8 hours a day, including class for 5 days a week, and 6 hours each for the other two days. The first four months were a trial period and we were scared to death lest we'd be dropped. But we were capped on schedule, and replaced our lightweight cuffs with stiff ones. I mention the cuffs because we were not permitted to remove them while on duty, and to give baths, clean utility rooms, etc. without getting them wet was a real challenge.

We lived in the Nurse's Residence and walked some distance to the buildings where we worked or ate. Our dining room was large, the nurses having tables of their own, and all ambulatory patients ate there also. The food was good and there was plenty of it. The grounds were planted with shrubs and flowers and were beautiful.

Trudeau was something like a private club and we all grew to love it, patients as well as nurses. It was located on the side of Mt. Pisgah and had a lovely view. The snow got pretty deep sometimes, and the temperatures dropped to 20 below, and not infrequently to 30 below. There were no windows, just screens on the biggest part of our sleeping porches, and the beds couldn't be brought inside. To go out and jump into a cold bed in below zero weather was hard to take.

The 23 months we spent at Trudeau flew by, and then we went to New York City to affiliate for three months at the Manhattan Maternity Hospital. The course was excellent but the hours and

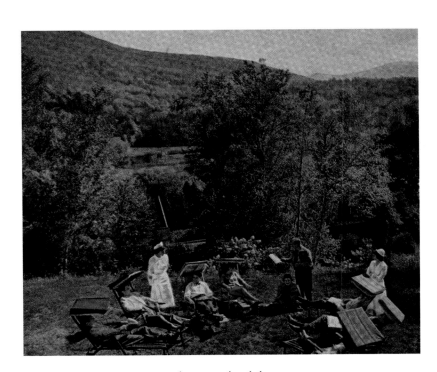

Nursing on the grounds of the sanatorium

*living conditions were not very desirable. . . .
Then I began my 10 months' affiliation with
Yale University School of Nursing where I
began my work on Surgical Pediatrics. I had
often thought I'd like to be a pediatric nurse,
but with brain tumors, ruptured appendices
(we didn't have antibiotics then and the
children often died), a baby badly burned,
and a few other heart-breaking cases, I
changed my mind.*

*After State Boards, I went to Trudeau where
I became Night Supervisor for a year. My
strongest recollection of this period was the
beautiful aurora borealis I saw many nights
after midnight, especially during the winter,
as I made my rounds to the various
buildings.*[26]

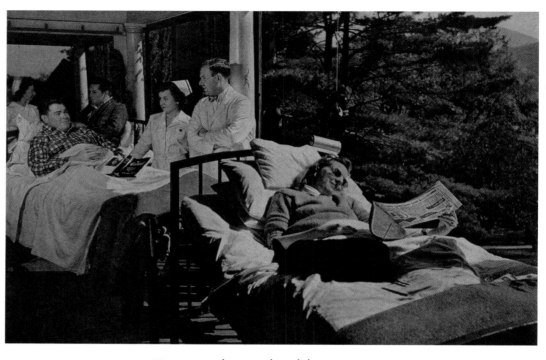

Nursing on the verandas of the sanatorium
Used with permission of "Saturday Evening Post" ©1951 (renewed BFL and MS Inc.)

Elizabeth left the sanatorium in 1937. She later obtained her bachelor's and master's degrees in nursing from Columbia University in New York City. Subsequently, in New York, she became Director of Nursing Service at Albany Medical Center, Director of the Russell Sage College School of Nursing, and Professor of Nursing on the Albany Medical College faculty. Elizabeth lived to be ninety-four, passing away on November 1, 1994.

All of the retired nurses who were interviewed prior to the writing of this book were asked to recall a story, one they would never forget, about caring for or living with one of the patients while at Trudeau Sanatorium. Their stories were sometimes humorous, often sad, but always touching.

The one thing that stood out when I first went to Trudeau was a fellow patient. We were assigned tables when we went to the dining room. I sat by a young man by the name of Henry Yee, a young Chinese fellow in his early twenties. He was about my age, probably. Henry sort of had a crush on me. He would come down to my cottage on Sunday morning and make sure that I went to church. If I wasn't up he would throw gravel at my window. He was the sweetest guy. He went for an x-ray one day and his TB had spread so he had to go back to the infirmary. The girls came around and taught him how to knit and crochet and stuff he could do by hand to keep him busy. When I would go to see him, if he didn't know I was coming, I'd see him stick his knitting down under the covers so I wouldn't see what he was doing. Why I'm telling you this — he died. And that I had never forgotten. You just didn't expect someone young like that to die. It was rough, very rough.[27]

I had a Cuban patient once. He was about thirty-eight years old. He was very, very wealthy. He had a wedding up here for a niece. He had a red carpet all the way from the church to the hotel. The whole town was invited. It was unbelievable — the money. And he said to me one time, "You know, I would give every bit of money I have if I could have your health." It really made an impression on me when I was eighteen. He said, "You don't know what it is to be devastated by disease." I think he died about ten or fifteen years later. That always stayed with me in my mind.[28]

TB defined our lives. Working with TB we felt we were collaborators. We felt we were doing what the great Dr. Edward Livingston Trudeau initiated. So we were members of an army in the fight against tuberculosis.[29]

I'll never forget one winter in Saranac Lake. The temperature was fifty degrees below zero. My assignment was to care for a male TB patient, twenty-five-years-old, critically ill in an oxygen tent on a twenty-hour private duty basis. I was to sleep on the porch adjoining his room, get up frequently during the night to give him hypos, etc. I was given three hours off during the day. The sum of six dollars per day was the amount received in compensation. The other nurses wrapped me up well with several wool sweaters, socks, scarf, knitted cap, and wool robe.

The patient informed me that I didn't look as bad as my three predecessors and that he would consider keeping me. This should have cheered me up but I have never experienced such cold in my life. I was twenty-three. The icicles were about one foot wide and extended the length of the window on the sleeping out porch. The only warm spot in the bed was where the small hot water heating unit was placed. There was no danger of going into a sound sleep and not hearing the patient's bell.

However, looking out the window, the night scene resembled a fairyland of lights . . . with sparkling white snow and ice. It was very beautiful.

The patient lasted only six weeks despite the best of care. I had to get another nurse to cover the night shift, as it was impossible to cover days and nights and stay awake. . . . I looked forward to finally closing my eyes without responsibility. I had lost sixteen pounds in six weeks — a hard way to do it.

After sleeping in an adjoining room for about an hour, the night nurse came to inform me that the patient had died.

I felt terrible! As soon as I turned his care over to another nurse he died. Later, when I fell into a deep sleep, the patient came to me in my dreams and told me that he was OK; that it had been time for him to go, and he assured me that I had done my best.

I awoke completely relieved. It was so realistic that it made me feel so much better. I am not a superstitious person but this experience will not be forgotten.

This was one of the more difficult cases of Dr. Francis Trudeau, Sr., who was a brilliant, kind, and understanding man. This experience was my only claim to fame.[30]

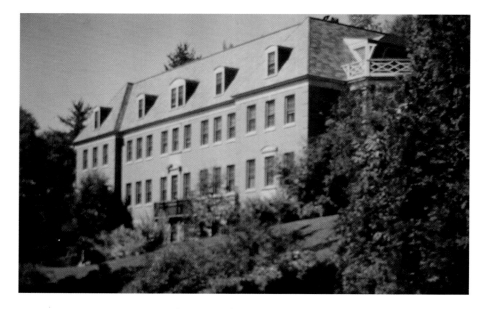

Reid House, the nurses' residence
Courtesy of the Trudeau Institute Archives

I was born in Goeppingen, Southern Germany, on May 9, 1921. When Hitler came to power in 1933, I was twelve years old. When I was a child, my dolls were either sick or in school. Although most of my friends had doll kitchens, I had a doll hospital given to me by my grandmother. For as long as I can remember I also loved to perform and dress up.

My parents, not yet wanting to leave Germany, had a house built in Stuttgart where I took a three-month certificate course in massage therapy. This course helped me later with my nursing. During my nursing days, backrubs were very important, especially in TB nursing where the patients had to be on complete bed rest. To this day, I believe in the therapeutic effect of massage.

I eventually emigrated to England but was restless there. I wanted to do something important with my life that would help those affected by the war. I decided to become a nurse and work in the slums of London so that I could take care of those people who had the greatest needs. Ultimately I was accepted at a very fine hospital, which was then called St. Alfege's.

The beautiful Nurse's Residence where we stayed was up the hill in Blackheath near Greenwich Park. Our nurse's training lasted four years and was very rigorous. We worked twelve-hour shifts. I did night duty there, and quite early in my training, I was in charge of forty male patients. After night duty, we had lectures by nurses and doctors.

I was frequently sent to work in Jenner, the tuberculosis ward. It was there that I witnessed my first death and that my fear of TB began. Although constant bombing surrounded me, I recall being more afraid of catching TB than of being killed by a bomb.

Nurses on day duty had to take turns sleeping in an air raid shelter at the hospital at night. We called it "Sleeping at the Dugout." Those were the only times we had to go into a shelter.

We were on call for casualties, of which there were many since Greenwich was in a badly bombed area. We had to keep the hospital as empty as possible so that we could take in new casualties.

Despite the rigor of the training and the frequent hardships we often endured, I managed to earn distinction for my training and was so honored at County Hall at Westminster.

Finally, the war ended.

My father and brother who had emigrated to the United States wanted me to join them there. While waiting for my visa I worked at St. Charles Hospital. Again I was sent to the TB ward and again the fear of tuberculosis gripped me. When I asked for a transfer to another ward, the matron refused. She said, "Nurse, I hope if you ever get TB nobody will want to nurse you." Those words came back to haunt me more than once.

When my visa finally arrived in March of 1946, I emigrated to America. Three weeks after arriving I began working at New York Hospital.

I was eventually assigned to TB patients. My fear of TB increased more and more. In the TB wards in England the windows were open and we were told that cross ventilation was very important. However, at New York Hospital the windows stayed shut.

I had a hard time adjusting to the big city of New York and to New York Hospital. I felt tired and frustrated. The slow elevator to the twelfth floor frustrated me. The closed windows on the TB ward frustrated me. The glamorous nurses frustrated me. During the seven long war years I had worn the same uniforms and not bought any clothes. So, when I compared myself to my nursing colleagues, I felt dowdy.

Then one day I spat up a little blood. Soon it was happening with relative frequency. My greatest fear was realized. I knew I had TB! I went to the infirmary and told the doctor of my fears. She seemed incredulous and called me a hypochondriac; a word I had never heard before. Was I really a hypochondriac and only imagining that I was spitting blood? Intuitively, I knew that I had TB and was most likely spreading it all over the hospital! But as no one believed me, back to work I went.

During the fall of 1948, after I had been in America for two years, I caught a cold. Because I was coughing so much I was finally x-rayed. Almost immediately, I was summoned back to the infirmary and there it was finally confirmed—I had TB. I guess I was not prepared to hear the words that confirmed what I already knew, because I still remember the shock I felt upon hearing that dreaded diagnosis. I thought, "Now I am going to die like all the patients back at St. Alfeges on Jenner Ward. I am going to die, and just like the Matron at St. Charles said, no one will want to nurse me because I didn't like to do TB nursing." I thought my life was over. There would be no more boyfriends; no husband, no children, no future.

Back I went to the TB ward; this time not a nurse, but as a patient put on complete bed rest. I remained tired, had lost my appetite, and was losing weight. Everybody brought me food but I just kept losing weight.

Despite all this, I kept getting worse. I had a cavity in my right lung. There was no pain, however, and it felt good not to have to do anything; to give in to this constant tiredness. I was also relieved that I was not a hypochondriac and that I was no longer spreading my TB to everyone I came in contact with. Visitors had to wear masks. The nurses wore masks and gowns but the windows stayed shut!

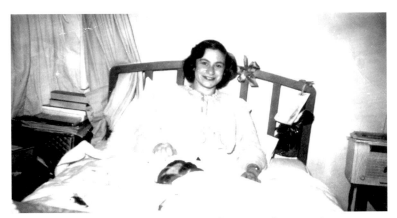

Lilo in bed on TB floor at New York Hospital, November 1948
Courtesy of Lilo Levine

While I was on the TB ward at New York Hospital, my primary nurse was from Saranac Lake where Trudeau Sanatorium was. She told me that the people at Trudeau were happy and that they got well.

My doctor, the one who had not believed that I had TB, came to see me several times. I think she was feeling guilty because she put in a lot of effort to get me into Trudeau.

I was taken to Grand Central Station and, by wheelchair, to the overnight train for Saranac Lake. I arrived there in February of 1949. I smelled the air; how delicious, how clear, and how clean it was. When we drove through the Trudeau gates my fear of TB and my fear of dying vanished! I fell in love with what I saw from the first moment. I was put on complete bed rest in Ludington Infirmary, one of the two infirmaries for the sickest patients.

My bed was wheeled out onto the porch. What a joy for me to have open windows at last! I was entranced with the glorious view of the mountains. And I did not mind the cold at all. We had electric blankets to keep us warm even when the temperature went to thirty below.

The progress of my recovery was as follows:

March 11, 1949: I had pneumonolysis which involved cutting of adhesions, which were preventing the lung from collapsing sufficiently with the pneumothorax treatment. This procedure was done at the Saranac Lake Hospital, which is now the Main building for North Country Community College.

March 17, St. Patrick's Day: My x-ray showed that my cavity had closed.

March 24: I had planograms which were images of different layers in the lungs. By then I had gained weight. I was now up to 107 pounds

March 26: I progressed to bathroom privileges still weighing 107 pounds.

April 1: My sputum was negative. We had our sputum tested regularly for the TB bacillus.

April 2: I finally got to self-care, which meant that I could go the bathroom and wash myself. That was a big day!

April 8: I weighed 108 pounds and got my first pass. This meant I could ride the Trudeau bus into town.

April 25: I moved to Gillender, which was a rest cottage. Here we were on bed rest but were allowed up for the meals that were delivered to the cottage. We were also allowed bathroom

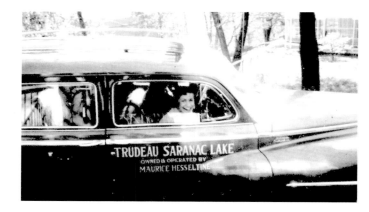

Lilo in the Trudeau Bus
Courtesy of Lilo Levine

privileges. We were on the porch day and night but had our meals in the living room. My favorite cottage mate was Ramphi Tulerak, from Siam. She was small like me, and we did a lot of giggling together. We took art classes from an instructor who came to the cottage.

April 28: My weight had gone up to 112 pounds.

May 19: I had more planograms. Refills for pneumothorax continued weekly.

June 6: An x-ray showed the cavity still closed.

June 16: I was able to start exercise, which meant I was allowed a five-minute walk once a day.

June 20: I was allowed to exercise five minutes twice a day.

June 27: I was allowed to exercise five minutes in the mornings and ten minutes in the afternoons.

June 28: My x-ray was still OK. I remember always worrying when I had an x-ray taken that I may have had a relapse. It was something that happened to other people but never to me.

August 6: I had my first meal in the dining room in the Main Building. This was a big event. On the first day in the dining room we were assigned a seat. Meals were served to us and were always very good.

August 16: I moved to Moore Cottage, which was an up cottage. Here we were allowed to get out of bed and go out whenever we wanted to. There were four of us in Moore Cottage who shared a bedroom and the porch. We still took rest hour every afternoon and continued to sleep on the porch with our electric blankets no matter how cold it got. There was a living room with a fireplace. We fixed our own breakfast on Sundays and had lots of fun parties.

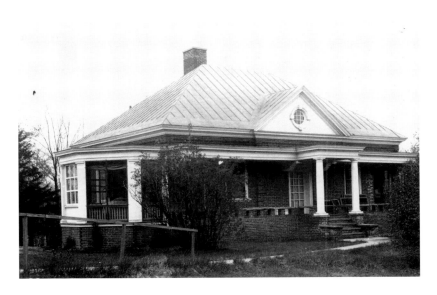

Moore Cottage
Courtesy of Lilo Levine

Some of the friendships I made at Moore Cottage have been friendships for life. There were Gretchen, Grace, and Melba. Then there was Cathy, who was also a nurse, and one year younger than I. Cathy had trained in Ireland while I trained in England. She came to New York with her sister and worked as a nurse in New York, where she also got TB. We are still very close friends. Then there was Edith who was married to Bill. When he came to visit he would build us a fire in the living room and take us for long rides in his car. Bill stuck by Edith, but not everyone was as fortunate. Many spouses were afraid of TB.

Then there was delightful Betty who was a young mother that had to leave her two little children because of her TB. Her husband and her mother took over the care of the children. How hard it was for her. I used to tease her and say, "Just think of all the diapers you don't have to change." Betty and her husband visited us here in Saranac Lake in 1999. What a treat! In spite of her worries about her young family, her memories of Trudeau, like mine, were fond ones.

Peggy was also one of our cottage mates who was in love with Joe, a patient at Sunmount Veteran's Hospital. Peggy and Joe were married in Saranac Lake in the fall of 1950. Betty and I were Peggy's bridesmaids.

On October 17, 1949 I started working one hour a day as a nurse on the grounds. I was back in my white uniform. It felt wonderful! I stopped keeping records. I gradually increased my nursing hours and loved working on the grounds. I loved TB nursing!!!

What follows was a typical workday for me on the grounds:

I reported to the Medical Building. Upstairs were treatment rooms and doctors' offices where pneumothorax was administered and patients were weighed. Keeping records of weight was important as a weight loss might mean a relapse. I don't ever recall any overweight patients despite all the rich food we ate.

After reporting for duty, I picked up my assignment sheet and checked what rest cottages I was assigned to. Then I prepared the syringes with the streptomycin, which was the main drug at the time for battling TB. Eventually a wooden box was designed especially for me so that I could

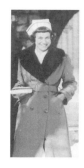

Delivering strepto
Courtesy of Lilo Levine

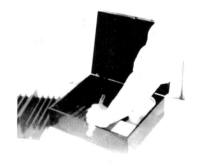

Carrier for streptomycin syringes
Courtesy of Lilo Levine

carry these syringes from cottage to cottage more easily. A picture of the box was later published in a nursing journal. I went on my way wearing my white uniform from New York Hospital and my graduate nurse's cap.

Often I was assigned to Kerbs I and Kerbs II, which were the male rest cottages. They were my favorite cottages right from the beginning. Maybe I sensed the good things that were looming on the horizon! I climbed the long snowy hill that led to the Kerbs cottages carrying my wooden box filled with streptomycin syringes. I made the beds, changed the beds on linen day, gave back rubs, talked with the patients, and helped pack up their belongings when they moved to an up cottage.

Whenever a new Jewish patient arrived at Trudeau, the Jewish Sisterhood sent a plant. One day, I had a phone call from one of the ladies, who said, "A nice young Jewish boy has arrived in Kerbs I. Would you like to take him a plant?" So I went up to Kerbs I on my day off and found what I thought was that nice Jewish boy and started giving him the plant. He said, "You don't want me. You want Melvin over there."

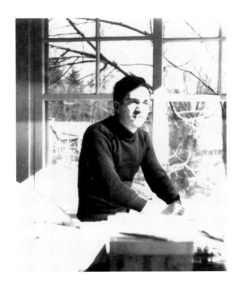

Mel Levine at Trudeau Sanatorium
Courtesy of Lilo Levine

And there was Melvin! He was lying flat on his back looking at me with his big bluish green eyes. He says they are blue but I see a touch of green in them. We started talking; I think the conversation was mostly about music. In the days to follow, I took care of Mel's bed and gave him back rubs. Looking back on those days, I'm convinced the head nurse knew what she was doing right from the start when she kept assigning me to Mel's cottage.

Soon Mel was allowed his first meal in the dining room. His cottage mates arranged for Mel to sit next to me. Then he was allowed his five-minute walk and we walked together and talked together. He was allowed more and more exercise, and we walked and talked more together.

Our favorite walk was on Trudeau Road, in those days called Smith Road, which had a beautiful view of the mountains. There was a big rock at the end of one of the driveways. As time went on, we spent many memorable hours sitting on that rock talking about absolutely everything.

Soon Mel moved to Phoenix, an up cottage for men. Phoenix is one of the few cottages that has not yet been torn down. By September, our friendship had grown into love. On Rosh Hashanah morning, before going to synagogue, we went out to the rock, which by now had become "Our Rock." This is where Mel asked me to marry him. A cloud lifted and the world suddenly seemed so bright and beautiful and clear.

We were married on December 31, 1950, in Saranac Lake at the Jewish Center. My good friend, Cathy, was at the wedding as were many of the nurses and doctors from Trudeau. After our wedding, we left Trudeau and moved to 12 Depot Street, where we had rented a furnished apartment. I continued nursing on the grounds and Mel worked part time at one of the Trudeau labs.

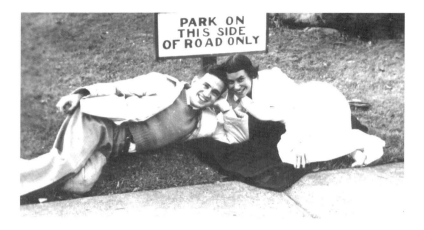

Mel and Lilo--"Cousins" at last!
Courtesy of Lilo Levine

When Mel had a relapse, after we were both discharged from Trudeau, he was given streptomycin and paraminosalacylic acid (PAS). It came in big white pills and I marveled that he had no problem swallowing this awful stuff. Mel stayed at home and rested and took PAS, and I continued working on Grounds until Mel was better. In May of 1952, we moved to Charlottesville, Virginia. Two years later Trudeau closed.

We moved back to Saranac Lake thirteen years ago when Mel retired from Brookhaven National Lab, where he was a Senior Scientist. I did not go back to nursing though many times I intended to.

Now it is fifty years since we were married. We celebrated our golden anniversary on New Years Eve, 2000, with our children and grandchildren at the Hotel Saranac.

TB and Trudeau—I can think of them both with love.

Written by Lilo Levine
Saranac Lake, New York, January 2001

The End of an Era

By the end of 1946, more than 15,000 patients had been treated at the sanatorium. However, due to the success of the various drug treatments for tuberculosis that were increasingly available, sanatoriums across the country began closing their doors. In November of 1954, the gates at Trudeau Sanatorium closed for the last time. Bea Sprague Edward remembers that day well.

All along everyone would say, "Oh Trudeau, that will go on forever. It will never close." Suddenly Dr. Francis Trudeau, Sr., dropped the bombshell. We were all called to a meeting. I can remember I was assisting with a pneumothorax down in one of the rooms when the call came in. "There is an emergency meeting, stop all pneumos, stop everything and come to the recreation hall." And when we heard the news of the closing we were stunned. Right after lunch, while the patients were resting, there was only one thought in my mind. I had to drive down to St. John's in the Wilderness and visit Dr. E. L. Trudeau's grave. When I got there I just stood there and said, "Look what's happened!" I needed to go talk to him. I just couldn't think of what else to do.

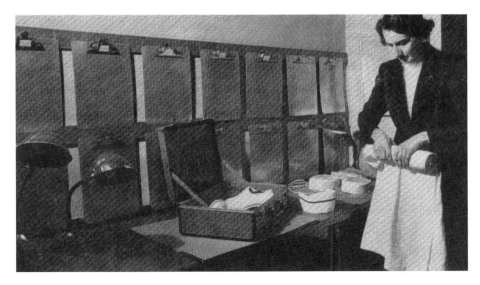

Marie Miller packing up the nurse's uniforms in 1954
Fritz Goro/Timepix

Marie Miller and I were the last ones left. We had to close up Ludington Infirmary — everything else was closed up then. "Life Magazine" came to take some pictures. The photographer went into the dark room in the X-ray Department and accidentally exposed a roll of film. That just seemed too cruel. Although he did get some pictures, the best ones were destroyed. The patients were gone, the place was empty, and those pictures never saw the light of day.[3]

Trudeau

You had to learn the great lesson alone
Ere you published plain truths to mankind;
To you our commonplace facts were unknown
And you blazed a new trail and outlined
A plan so straightforward, so simple so plain
At first it was hard to believe
That rest, air and food made the tripod of gain
For those who lost health would retrieve.

You lighted the torch, O bold pioneer!
And your torch soon gave place to a lamp
With oil of courage, persistence and cheer,
And it lighted a world to your camp.
From your fires, Adirondack, we've taken
   our glow,
You taught us to cast away fear;
May we ever thy watchword re-echo, Trudeau!
Thy spirit of progress lives here.
             ~G. E. May, MD

Introduction

[1] (Identification and Management of Tuberculosis, May 2000)

Definitions of Terms

[1] (The Trudeau Institute: A Century of Science, 1984)
[2] (Trudeau, 1899, p. 145)

Chapter 1

[1] (Bruno, December 31, 1999)
[2] (Krause, 1917, p. 295)
[3] (Bruno, December 31, 1999)
[4] (Trudeau, 1915, p. 12)
[5] (Trudeau, 1915, pp. 9-10)
[6] (Trudeau, 1915, pp.10)
[7] (Trudeau, 1915, pp. 13)
[8] (Trudeau, 1915, pp. 10-11)
[9] (Krause, 1925, p. 18)
[10] (Trudeau, 1915, p. 15)
[11] (Trudeau, 1915, p. 26)
[12] (Trudeau, 1915, pp. 27-28)
[13] (Dock and Stewart, 1920)
[14] (Trudeau, 1915, p. 31)
[15] (Trudeau, 1915, p. 32)
[16] (Trudeau, 1915, p. 38)
[17] (Trudeau, 1915, pp. 38-39)
[18] (Trudeau, 1915, p. 40)
[19] (Trudeau, 1915, pp. 71-72)
[20] (Trudeau, 1915, p. 78)
[21] (Caldwell, 1988, p. 42)
[22] (Trudeau, 1915, pp. 80-81)
[23] (Trudeau, 1915, p. 89)

[24] (Murray, 1989, pp. 11-13)
[25] (Trudeau, 1915, pp. 97-98)
[26] (Trudeau, 1915, p. 100)
[27] (Trudeau, 1915, p. 101)
[28] (Smith, 1910, p. 175)
[29] (Editor, 1910, p. 159)
[30] (Trudeau, 1915, p. 106)
[31] (Trudeau, 1915, pp. 108-109)
[32] (Trudeau, 1915, p. 150)
[33] (Trembley, 1910, p. 174)
[34] (Trudeau, 1915, p. 154)
[35] (Trudeau, 1915, p. 155)
[36] (Trudeau, 1915, pp. 165-166)
[37] (Trudeau, 1915, p. 84)
[38] (Trudeau, 1915, p. 168)
[39] (Trudeau, 1915, p. 170)
[40] (Lindsay, 1925, pp. 44-45)
[41] (Trudeau, 1915, pp. 173-174)
[42] (Krause, 1925, p. 13)
[43] (Trudeau, 1915, p. 205)
[44] (Trudeau, 1915, p. 194)
[45] (Biggs, 1910, p. 163)
[46] (Krause, 1925, pp. 19-20)
[47] (Trudeau, 1915, p. 244)
[48] (Trudeau, 1915, p. 221)

[49] (Williams, 1925 p. 54)
[50] (White, 1954, p. 174)
[51] (Goldthwaite, 1915, p. 8)
[52] (Trudeau, 1915, pp. 220, 231)
[53] (Trudeau, 1915, pp. 231, 232)
[54] (Krause, 1925)
[55] (Trudeau, 1915, pp. 235, 237)
[56] (Trudeau, 1915, pp. 181-82)
[57] (Trudeau, 1915, p. 251)
[58] (Trudeau, 1915, p. 283)
[59] (Trudeau, cited in Ellison, 1994, p. 153)
[60] (Gallos, 1985, p. 6)
[61] (Trudeau, 1915, pp. 286-287)
[62] (Trudeau, 1915, pp. 271-273)
[63] (Trudeau, 1915, p. 275)
[64] (Trudeau, 1915, pp. 276-277)
[65] (Trudeau, 1915, pp. 310-312)
[66] (Trudeau, 1915, pp. 300-301)
[67] (Krause 1925, p. 16)
[68] (Scrapbook 10)
[69] (Scrapbook 10)
[70] (Editor, 1956)
[71] (Altman, 1995)
[72] (Altman, 1995)
[73] (Looking for the cure, 2000)

Chapter 2

1. (White, 1951)
2. (Trudeau, 1915, p. 172)
3. (Caldwell, 1988)
4. (Dickens, cited in Dormandy, 2000, p. 92)
5. (Caldwell, 1988, p. 50)
6. (1887 Annual Report)
7. (1897-98 Annual Report)
8. (Trudeau, cited in Ellison, 1994, p. 162)
9. (Trudeau, cited in Ellison, 1994, p. 152)
10. (J. Gage, personal communication, July 5, 1995.)
11. (Krause, 1925, p. 11)
12. (Caldwell, 1988, p. 74)
13. (Brown, 1913, p. 478)
14. (Scrapbook 8)
15. (Brown, 1925, p. 25)
16. (Quiroga, 1995, p. 40)
17. (Quiroga, 1995)
18. (Quiroga, 1995, p. 13)
19. (Johnson, 1907, pp. 134-135)
20. (Trudeau, 1904)
21. (Editor, 1904)
22. (Brown, 1925, p. 27)
23. (Baldwin, 1916, p. 33)
24. (Trudeau, cited in Teller, 1988, p. 55)
25. (Teller, 1988, p. 82)
26. (Brown, 1916)
27. (Brown, 1908)
28. (Somerfield, 1914)
29. (Gallos, 1985, pp. 25-26)
30. (Baldwin, 1925)
31. (Smith, 1909, p. 407)
32. (E. Montalbine, personal communication, July 26, 1995)
33. (L. Levine, personal communication, November 26, 1999)
34. (Kernan, 1904)
35. (Smith, 1909, p. 409)
36. (Brown, 1916, pp. 61-62)
37. (Brown, 1916, pp. 20-50)
38. (Brown, 1916, p. 73)
39. (Gallos, 1985)
40. (W, F.N., 1906, pp. 371-372)
41. (Brown, 1916, p. 74)
42. (L. Levine, personal communication, November 26, 1999)
43. (I. Mushlin, personal communication, January 11, 2001)
44. (Caldwell, 1988)
45. (E. Montalbine, personal communication, July 26, 1995)
46. (P. McLaughlin, personal communication, July 5, 1995)
47. (J. McNeil, personal communication, July 5, 1995)
48. (Trudeau, 1910)
49. (Kernan, 1904, p. 26)
50. (Smith, 1909, pp. 407-408)
51. (Anonymous, 1910, pp. 68-69)
52. (Dyer, 1919, p. 335)
53. (Schaeffer, 1935)
54. (Scrapbook 11)
55. (Taylor, 1986, p. 148)
56. (Brown, 1916, pp. 44-47)
57. (I. Mushlin, personal communication, January 11, 2001)
58. (Brown, 1916, pp. 47-49)
59. (Caldwell, 1988, p. 119)
60. (McLaughlin, cited in Caldwell, 1988, p. 131)
61. (Hines, 1946, p.75)
62. (B. Edward, personal communication, January 15, 2001)
63. (Anonymous, 1904)
64. (Gallos, 1985, p. 31)
65. (C. Pendergast, personal communication, February 20, 2001)
66. (Hotaling, cited in Robinson, 1987)
67. (Adirondack Daily Enterprise, cited in Dalton, 1930)
68. (vonArdyn, cited in Dalton, 1930)
69. (Davis, 1927)

Chapter 3

1. (Donahue, 1996, p. 191)
2. (Dock & Stewart, 1920)
3. (Donahue, 1996, pp. 195,197)
4. (Robinson, cited in Donahue, 1996, p. 197)
5. (Nightingale, 1860))
6. (Dock & Stewart, 1920)
7. (Nightingale, cited in Donahue, 1996, p. 275)
8. (Wolf, cited in Donahue, 1996, p. 307)
9. (Box 2, File 208)
10. (Gallos, 1985)
11. (Burgess, 1925, p. 41)
12. (Kernan, 1904, pp. 25-27)
13. (Smith, 1909, pp. 407-409)
14. (Baldwin, 1925)
15. (Burnett, 1919)
16. (Box 4, File 1265)
17. (1911 Annual Report)
18. (Box 4, File 1265)
19. (1913 Annual Report)
20. (Scrapbook on D. Ogden Mills School of Nursing)
21. (Scrapbook on D. Ogden Mills School of Nursing)
22. (Scrapbook on D. Ogden Mills School of Nursing)
23. (Scrapbook on D. Ogden Mills School of Nursing)
24. (Bell, 1980, p. 5)
25. (Bell, 1980, p. 7)
26. (Bell, 1980, pp. 8-10)
27. (E. Montalbine, personal communication, July 26, 1995)
28. (J. Gage, personal communication, June 25, 1996)
29. (I. Mushlin, personal communication, January 11, 2001)
30. (E. Healy, personal communication, June 25, 1996)
31. (B. Edward, personal communication, January 15, 2001)

1887 Annual Report. In *Trudeau Sanatorium Annual Reports*, 1897-1927. Saranac Lake: Trudeau.

1897-98 Annual Report. In *Trudeau Sanatorium Annual Reports*, 1897-1927. Saranac Lake: Trudeau.

1911 Annual Report. In *Trudeau Sanatorium Annual Reports*, 1885-1895,1897-1927. Saranac Lake: Trudeau.

1913 Annual Report. In *Trudeau Sanatorium Annual Reports*, 1885-1895,1897-1927. Saranac Lake: Trudeau.

Box 2, File 208. Trudeau, E. L. 1908. Farewell Speech to Miss Collins. In Adirondack Collection, Saranac Free Library.

Box 4, File 1265. Reid, E. M. In Adirondack Collection, Saranac Free Library.

Identification and Management of Tuberculosis 2001. [Web Page]. American Academy of Family Physicians May 2000 [cited February 14 2001]. Available from http://aafp.org/afp/2000050/2667.html.

Looking for the cure. Trudeau Institute [cited 2000 October 10]. Available from http://www.trudeauinstitute.org/info/history/history.htm.

Scrapbook 8. From a series of Scrapbooks containing clippings about the Adirondack Cottage Sanitarium. Saranac Lake, NY: Trudeau Institute Library.

Scrapbook 10. From a series of Scrapbooks containing clippings about the Adirondack Cottage Sanitarium. Saranac Lake, NY: Trudeau Institute Library.

Scrapbook 11. From a series of Scrapbooks containing clippings about the Adirondack Cottage Sanitarium. Saranac Lake, NY: Trudeau Institute Library.

Scrapbook on D. Ogden Mills School of Nursing. From a series of Scrapbooks containing clippings about the Adirondack Cottage Sanitarium. Saranac Lake, NY: Trudeau Institute Library.

Altman, L. K. 1995. "Francis B. Trudeau, 75, Founder of Biological Research Institute." *The New York Times*.

Anonymous. 1904. "'Cousining' Once, But, Etc." *Journal of the Outdoor Life* 1 (1).

Anonymous. 1910. "The Daily Round: The Patient's Viewpoint, One of Optimism and Cheerfulness." *Journal of the Outdoor Life* VII (3):68-69.

Baldwin, E. R. 1916. "The Trudeau School of Tuberculosis." *Journal of the Outdoor Life* XIII (2): 33-34.

Baldwin, E. R. 1925. "The Trudeau Sanatorium Anniversary." *Journal of the Outdoor Life* XXII (1):7-10.

Bell, E. A. 1980. "A history of my life." In *Adirondack Collection*, Saranac Lake Free Library. Saranac Lake.

Biggs, H. M. 1910. "Dr. Trudeau as a Pioneer in the Antituberculosis Movement." *Journal of the Outdoor Life* VII (7):163-165.

Brown, L. 1908. *The Sanatorium*. Eighteenth Series ed. Vol. 1, International Clinics. Philadelphia: J. B. Lipincott Company.

Brown, L. 1913. *The Symptoms, Diagnosis, Prognosis, Prophylaxis and Treatment of Tuberculosis*. Edited by W. Osler and T. McCrae, Modern Medicine in Theory and Practice. Philadelphia: Lea and Febiger.

Brown, L. 1916. *Rules for Recovery from Tuberculosis*. New York: Lea & Febiger.

Brown, L. 1925. "Personal Reflections." *Journal of the Outdoor Life* XXII (1):22-27.

Bruno, J. December 31, 1999. "Dr. Edward Trudeau: Cornerstone of a Community." *Adirondack Daily Enterprise*, December 31, 1999, 3.

Burnett, G. M. 1919. "The Tuberculosis Nurse." *Journal of the Outdoor Life* XVI (2):48-49.

Caldwell, M. 1988. *The last crusade: The war on consumption*, 1862-1954. New York: Atheneum.

Dalton, J. T. 1930. *Land of Dreams and Other Poems*. New York: The Knickerbocker Press.

Davis, R. H. "The Story of a Great Heart That Dared Not Beat Too Fast," *The New York Sun*, October 20, 1927.

Dock, L. L., and I. M. Stewart. 1920. *A Short History of Nursing*. 4th ed. New York: G. P. Putnum's Sons.

Donahue, M. P. 1996. *Nursing, The Finest Art: An Illustrated History*. 2nd ed. St. Louis: Mosby.

Dormandy, T. 2000. *The White Death: A History of Tuberculosis*. New York: New York University Press.

Dyer, E. S. 1919. "The Psychology of Saranac." *Journal of the Outdoor Life* VI (11):334-335.

Editor. 1904. "The Outdoor Life." *The Outdoor Life* I (1):1.

Editor. 1910. "Edward Livingston Trudeau — A Biographical Sketch." *Journal of the Outdoor Life* VII (6):157-161.

Editor. 1956. "Dr. Francis." *Adirondack Daily Enterprise*, July 20, 1956, 5.

Ellison, D. L. 1994. *Healing Tuberculosis in the Woods: Medicine and Science at the End of the Nineteenth Century*, Contributions in medical studies no. 41. Westport, Conn.: Greenwood Press.

Gallos, P. L. 1985. *Cure Cottages of Saranac Lake: Architecture and History of a Pioneer Health Resort*. Saranac Lake, NY: Historic Saranac Lake.

Goldthwaite, K. W. 1915. "Dr. Edward Livingston Trudeau Died November 15, 1915." *The Adirondack Enterprise*, November 15, 1915.

Hines, D. P. 1946. *No Wind of Healing*. Garden City, New York: Doubleday & Co., Inc.

Johnson, H. 1907. "To While the Hours Away." *Journal of the Outdoor Life* IV (4):134-136.

Kernan, A. 1904. "Nursing at the Adirondack Cottage Sanitarium." *The Johns Hopkins Nurses, Alumni Magazine*:24-27.

Krause, A. K. 1917. "Edward L. Trudeau: A Study." *Journal of the Outdoor Life* XIV (10):295-297.

Krause, A. K. 1925. "Reflections on Doctor Trudeau." *Journal of the Outdoor Life* XXII (1):11-21.

Lindsay, C. P. 1925. "The Sanatorium in 1887." *Journal of the Outdoor Life* XXII (1):44-45.

Murray, W. H. H. 1989. *Adventures in Wildnerness*: Adirondack Museum and Syracuse University Press. Original edition, 1869.

Nightingale, F. 1860. *Notes on Nursing: What It Is and What It Is Not*. Dover Edition, unabridged republication of first American edition, ed. New York: D. Appleton and Company.

Quiroga, V. 1995. *Occupational Therapy: The first 30 Years*. MD: The American Occupational Therapy Association, Inc.

Robinson, R. 1987. "Reunion at Saranac Lake Stirs Memories for TB Patients." *The Post-Standard*, A-5(N).

Smith, M. 1909. "The Adirondack Cottage Sanitarium at Trudeau, NY." *The American Journal of Nursing* (March).

Smith, P. 1910. "Dr. Trudeau's First Winter in the Adirondacks." *Journal of the Outdoor Life* VII (6):175-176.

Somerfield, A. 1914. "The Adventures of T.B. Germ as Told by Himself." *Journal of the Outdoor Life* XI (4).

Taylor, R. 1986. *Saranac: America's Magic Mountain*. Boston: Houghton Mifflin.

Teller, M. E. (1988). *The Tuberculosis Movement: A Public Health Campaign in the Progressive Era*. New York: Greenwood Press.

The Trudeau Institute: A Century of Science. 1984. Saranac Lake, NY: The Trudeau Institute.

Trembley, C. C. 1910. "Dr. Trudeau as a Woodsman." *Journal of the Outdoor Life* VII (6):173-175.

Trudeau, E. L. (1899). "The Adirondack Cottage Sanitarium for the Treatment of Incipient Pulmonary Tuberchuosis." *The Practitioner* 62: 131-46.

Trudeau, E. L. 1904. "A Foreword from Dr. Trudeau." *Outdoor Life* 1 (1):1.

Trudeau, E. L. 1915. *An Autobiography*. Garden City, N.Y.: Lea & Febiger.

White, W. C. 1954. *Adirondack Country*. [1st] ed. New York,: Duell Sloan & Pearce.

Williams, H. L. 1925. "Stevenson and Trudeau." *Journal of the Outdoor Life* XXII (1):54-55.

W., F. N. 1906. "Sleeping Outdoors in Winter." *Journal of the Outdoor Life* III (10):369-372.

COUSINING: Romantic involvement between tuberculosis patients.

CURING: The process of bringing about a recovery from tuberculosis. Its usage implied that the person "curing" was a patient who lived in a TB sanatorium, institution, or cure cottage, throughout the duration of the cure, which could last weeks, months, or even years. Its usage does not imply that a cure actually took place, only that some form of treatment was in process. In other words, a patient who "cured" could later die of tuberculosis.

SANITARIUM VS. SANATORIUM: Although many think the terms "sanitarium" and "sanatorium" to be interchangeable, there is a semantic difference between the two words. "Sanitarium" is derived from the Latin word *sanitas*, which means health. In Dr. Trudeau's time, "sanitarium" was used in relation to all chronic care institutions. However, because of its close link with the word "sanity" it was often linked to institutions that treated mental disorders. "Sanatorium" comes from the Latin word *sanare*, which means to heal. Therefore, at the turn of the century it became the preferred word for the treatment of consumptives. After Dr. Trudeau's death, the Adirondack Cottage Sanitarium was renamed the Trudeau Sanatorium.[1] For the sake of continuity, this book will use the latter spelling of the word.

Surgical Treatments

ARTIFICIAL PNEUMOTHORAX: Collapse of the lung by the introduction of gas or filtered air into the chest cavity for the purpose of resting the diseased lung. Refills of air were first given every other day, then twice a week, once a week, once every two weeks, once a month, and finally every four to six weeks. Pneumothorax was to be continued for a period of from two to four or more years.

BILATERAL PNEUMOTHORAX: Compression of both lungs by pneumothorax. Actually, only a portion of both lungs was collapsed. Therefore, patients taking bilateral pneumothorax, though short of breath, could lead moderately active lives.

SURGICAL ALTERATION OF THE PHRENIC NERVE: Surgical compression or severing of the phrenic nerve was a treatment that attempted to rest the affected lung by disrupting the nerve innervations to the diaphragm. This was performed when other less drastic treatments failed to produce desired results.

THORACOPLASTY: Removal of the ribs on one side of the chest to accomplish a permanent collapse of the diseased part of that lung. This was considered only after other treatment modalities were deemed a failure.

Dr. Trudeau's Stages of Tuberculosis

INCIPIENT: Cases in which both the physical and rational signs point to slight local and constitutional involvement.

ADVANCED: Cases in which the localized disease process is either extensive or in an advanced state, or where, with a comparatively slight amount of pulmonary involvement, the rational signs point to grave constitutional impairment or to some complication.

FAR ADVANCED: Cases in which both the rational and physical signs warrant the term.

APPARENTLY CURED: Cases in which the rational signs of phthisis and the bacilli in the expectoration have been absent for at least three months, or who have no expectoration at all, any abnormal physical signs remaining being interpreted as indicative of a healed lesion.

ARRESTED: Cases in which cough, expectoration, and bacilli are still present, but in which all constitutional disturbance has disappeared for several months, the physical signs being interpreted as indicative of a retrogressive or arrested process.[2]